# PISS TO BLISS

# PISS TO BLISS

## Fed up With Cystitis, Chronic Bladder Pain & Women's Health Taboos Ruining Your Life?

Welcome to the Empowering
### HAPPY BLADDER BOOK

A multi-level approach, self-help guide on bladder health and breaking taboos that hold women back.

Get enlightened on Urinary Tract Infections UTI, Interstitial Cystitis IC, Sexual Cystitis, Candida/Thrush, Overactive Bladder OAB, Stress Urinary Incontinence SUI, IBS, Bladder Stones, Metaphysical Cystitis, Bladder Cancer, women's taboos and much more.

DR JENNIFER MEYER

First Edition. Published in 2019 by Dr J Meyer
www.drjmeyer.com

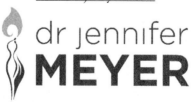

## Copyright and Disclaimer

**Copyright © 2019 by Dr Jennifer MEYER**

Piss to Bliss. Fed up with cystitis, chronic bladder pain & women's health taboos ruining your life? Welcome to the empowering Happy Bladder Book.

All rights reserved. No part of this publication including illustrations and meditations, may be reproduced, distributed or transmitted in any form or by any means, including photocopying, recording, or other electronic or mechanical methods, without the prior written permission of the publisher, except in the case of brief quotations embodied in critical reviews and certain other non-commercial uses permitted by copyright law.

Although the author and publisher have made every effort to ensure that the information in this book was correct at press time, the author and publisher do not assume and hereby disclaim any liability to any party for any loss, damage, or disruption caused by errors or omissions, whether such errors or omissions result from negligence, accident, or any other cause.

Adherence to all applicable laws and regulations, including international, federal, state and local governing professional licensing, business practices, advertising, and all other aspects of doing business in the US, Canada or any other jurisdiction is the sole responsibility of the reader and consumer.

Neither the author nor the publisher assumes any responsibility or liability whatsoever on behalf of the consumer or reader of this material. Any perceived slight of any individual or organization is purely unintentional.

The resources in this book are provided for informational purposes only and should not be used to replace the specialized training and professional judgment of a health care or mental health care professional.

Neither the author nor the publisher can be held responsible for the use of the information provided within this book. Please always consult a trained professional before making any decision regarding treatment of yourself or others.

**There are no medical claims made in this book. It is solely the opinion of the author.**

Paperback ISBN 978-1-9163122-0-3
Audio Format coming soon...
Also available as Amazon E-book: ASIN: B081B5H1KM

# Dedication

**This book is dedicated to the strong women in my family and beyond.**

Jackie Meyer (née Barham, my mama),

My grandmothers: Doris Barham (née King), & Ginette Meyer (née Paul).

My paternal great-grandmother, 'Mémé Lili', Athilie Paul (née Rahon), who suffered from cystitis all her life. I was unable to help her as I had not yet mastered my own bladder issues or written this book.

My maternal formidable great-grandmothers Jessie Kettle, Emma Exall, Emily Smith (my Guardian Angel), and Sarah Falkener – a suffragette in London whose courage helped to change the lives of women.

My paternal great-grandparents, including Anna Meyer (née Vogler) and other family members who formed part of 'la resistance' fighting the Nazis during the occupation in Paris.

All women from that era who didn't get the respect they deserved.

Thank you for your courage that gave us the voice we have today.

**To all those unsung heroes from the past, the present and the future: I salute you.**

# Your Free Gifts

When I go on a trip with a friend, I like to surprise her with a gift as we begin.

As a thank you for purchasing this book, here are some super-duper presents that I hope you will find useful.

1- Products & Services Reference. I have done the time-consuming research and linked them in one easy place: drjmeyer.com/free-gifts

2- Free webinar based on this book & introducing the *Piss to Bliss Online Course*: drjmeyer.com/free-gifts

3- Invitation to join The Happy Bladder Tribe, our private Facebook group: facebook.com/groups/497363147337943/

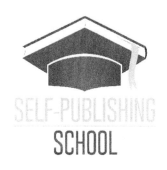

SELF-PUBLISHING
SCHOOL

# NOW IT'S YOUR TURN

**Discover the EXACT 3-step blueprint you need to become a bestselling author in 3 months.**

Self-Publishing School helped me, and now I want them to help you with this FREE WEBINAR.

Even if you're busy, bad at writing, or don't know where to start, you CAN write a bestseller and build your best life.

With tools and experience across a variety of niches and professions, Self-Publishing School is the <u>only</u> resource you need to take your book to the finish line!

**DON'T WAIT**

Watch this FREE WEBINAR now, and

Say "YES" to becoming a bestseller: (Advert)

**By clicking below on my affiliate link, you will get the best price available for joining. At the point of purchase mention my name to ensure your discount.**

**<u>bit.ly/35CQ4md</u>**

# Table of Contents

# PART ONE

## The WHYS
## As in the *wise* :o)

Understanding our Waterworks &
how bladder problems arise

We have now set our GPS coordinates for
Happy Bladder Land.

Start the road trip soundtrack...

# Warning

This book is written for women who have suffered regularly from cystitis, other bladder or urinary problems and wish to learn why it happens, how to stop it and are open-minded and ready to make some lifestyle changes.

We dive deep and some action steps are not conventional. I'm sharing my personal stories in my own voice, which is not always polite. I break taboos and don't shy away from embarrassing subjects such as toilets, cussing, recommending certain products, and sex; if it helps to understand cystitis, then I mention it without apology.

This book is a conversation with my best friend, it is not a medical consultation nor a university lecture.

- **Note to parents**: although all girls need to know about women's issues and how to avoid them, please be aware that this book is aimed at women of sexually active age. You may wish to black out the parts you deem unfit for your daughter to read, or just relay the important information relevant to her for her own health.

  I will be releasing an age-appropriate version of this book for young teenagers called, *Yip-Pee,* as I think it is important for girls of all ages to know how to look after themselves and to grow up with confidence about their bodies.

- **Note to Men**: high five, Dude, and welcome. I wrote this as if talking to my best girl however, men are allowed! Bladders affect both men and women. The information in this book will help you as well as the women in your life, so please don't be put off by the way it is written, dive in and get your nuggets of gold to help you on your own bladder journey.

\* \* \*

This book **is probably not** for you if you have never suffered from bladder pain or other women's inflammatory issues, are not prepared to make changes, are closed-minded, are expecting a medical or academic textbook, or if you take offence to swear-words, sexual content, straight-talking, vulnerable stories, product recommendations, or metaphysics.

You have been warned.

\* \* \*

# Introduction

Still with me? Awesome. Warning over, let's get into it.

My fascination with healing steered me to a PhD in Metaphysics, including natural health. I earned many diplomas and certifications in different holistic therapies and nutrition over the last three decades. I have put myself through the protocols shared within this book, and they worked for me, so now, I'd like to share my expertise and opinions with you.

I help women held back by ill-health and society's shackles to overcome health issues and break free from limitations and expectations. I empower them to create their most vibrant life. This book is the first in a women's health and empowerment series and mostly addresses urinary issues at *all* levels.

* * *

**Let's dive right in**

I understand: living with cystitis is at best, frustrating, and at worst, a death-wish.

*Bladder ills are unendurable agonies that ripple effect at many levels.*

You may be familiar with some of the following bladder related pains:

**Physical pain**

- Ranging from a mild ache to being knifed in the stomach.

- From holding your tummy to not being able to get up.

- Electrical charges clawing up the urethra into the bladder like having a dentist drill your tooth and hit a nerve.

- A dead butt imprinted with the toilet seat, after being stuck to it for an insufferable amount of time.

- Undeniable bladder cramps and erratic spasms that feels as if it is trying to give birth to itself.

- From a few drops of blood to frightening bleeding when you pee.

- The devastating need to go to the toilet all the time, only to squeeze out a few acid drops that burn.

- A stiff neck and back from uncontrollable bad posture and long-term agony.

- Eventually, a sore throat due to screaming, desperation and crying.

**Emotional and mental pain**

- The anguish the first sensation brings and the frustration as it develops: nothing else causes the irritability that cystitis does.

- You want to recoil as the world outside feels like it's prodding you with cattle sticks and sharp knives.

- The need to escape and the desire to shut yourself away in the dark.

- Stress, tears, frustration, shame, worry what others may think, and anger dominate your day.

- Dealing with taboos and misunderstandings around cystitis, especially the one that cystitis is a sexually transmitted disease and dirty: *it is not.*

### Relationship and sexual pain

- Friction caused by not wanting your partner coming near you.

- The agony of sex whilst having cystitis.

- Maybe you are single, as your partner had enough of your 'women troubles'.

- The thought of never wanting sex again, in case it makes you ill.

- Your sexual health and romantic life take a head-nose dive as cystitis leads the way *again* to despair.

- Arguments and tension with people, especially those who don't understand or sympathise at all, or worse, who belittle your pain.

- Colleagues avoid you as you turn from lovely-lady to narky-bitch and get the 'time of the month' label thrown at you.

- Family avoid you or comment flippantly 'Oh, no, it's the grumpy you '.

- Your self-confidence and self-love forever decrease.

- Feeling like a bad mother when you are unable to look after your children or snap at them as a result of chronic pain.

- Resentment of the 'you' that cystitis creates.

## Medical incompetence pain

- Paying good money to seek medical help and not getting satisfactory results.

- At best, doctors give you antibiotics that may or may not work, and at worst they tell you to get over it, go home and drink some cranberry juice. It is rare to find the desired support from the medical world.

- Hoping the General Practitioner (GP) will refer you this time to a urologist, then the devastation when they don't.

- Finally being referred only to be squished by the long waiting list.

- Finally seeing a specialist or paying for tests yourself that come back negative and you end up feeling like a fraud.

- Knowing there is something wrong with you but the doctors can't help you.

## Financial pain

- Finding the money to pay the huge bills for the urology tests.

- The cost of endless pricy painkillers, cranberry juice, cystitis sachets and other medications.

- Nobody pays you sick-leave if you are self-employed.

- Lost income for not being able to show up to work because you are, once again, sobbing on the toilet. How many hours have we spent off work with cystitis or bladder issues? How many wages or clients has it cost you?

- If you are employed, then the stress of providing endless doctors' notes that you are indeed suffering just about puts you over the edge. How about the loss of promotions or work travel due to your women health issues?

- What about that taboo that cystitis isn't really a big deal, making you feel you are 'pulling a sickie,' attention-seeking, or being a bit of a drama queen.

**Belief, frustration, victimhood pain**

- 'Why me? Not cystitis again! What am I doing wrong? Life isn't fair.'

- Down-spiral leading to many other negative issues in life.

- Fear of not knowing what to do to avoid cystitis.

- Loss of hope turning into chaos and desperation. If you reach that stage, it can permeate every part of your life, the pain of living with cystitis or the fear of getting it again becomes all-encompassing.

- Discomfort within yourself as self-judgement begins.

- Depression of your aura and energy frequency, dampening the real you and sucking you into a negative spiral, attracting people who do not understand, who may abuse you because you are weakened.

- Not defending yourself because of loss of self-esteem and self-confidence.

- Saying yes when you want to say no.

- Being *too nice* to make up for feeling so vulnerable inside.

- You may end up sometimes believing that you can't cope with your own life, or your ability to control your bladder.

- Cystitis has claimed its victim.

* * *

I hear you. I understand because I have been there too.

I've experienced the whole scale ranging from a mild cystitis lasting up to an hour, to when I needed a week off work with antibiotics, and then to the extreme of bleeding out from my bladder and consequently rushed to hospital for a transfusion and to clear a ravenous UTI e-coli infection that led to sepsis and nearly took my life.

I reached the point of preferring not waking up than living one more day with cystitis. After suffering all my life from my nemesis, it was time to turn this around once and for all or die: it was the catalyst for this book.

Publishing this book means it's the last chapter in my bladder suffering. Now, I want to offer you the same opportunity to help yourself.

*Why would you want to trust me with this important task?*

Well, because I have literally written the book.

I am now cystitis-free and it feels liberating, but it wasn't always that way.

I remember my first cystitis that I was aware of. I was four years old. I used to call it my 'funny tummy ache' and no one was able to help me as I couldn't explain it properly. I lived with cystitis or the fear of having it, all my life, up till now.

I've been hospitalised three times because of cystitis.

I had antibiotics for it *every month*, for years.

On my birthday in 2018, on a celebratory trip to Spain, I was lying in a foreign hospital fighting for my life, my wish was to never suffer again from bladder pain and if that meant not waking up, then so be it.

I asked my soul if we die tomorrow then do we have any regrets? That night I dreamed of this book and made myself a commitment: I will share my journey. If it means helping one woman never to have to be in my situation, it was worth writing.

I will show you actions steps to help yourself, covering several categories, including physical, mental, emotional, spiritual, nutritional, sexual, social and metaphysical.

As a result of what I share in this book, you may not only avoid cystitis but also find hope and the tools to change your life for the better.

*Let's see how joyful and adventurous your life can be without cystitis or the threat of ever having it again. Now, isn't that a welcome image?*

This is a functional, comprehensive, hand-holding guide to help bladder issues, a result of information that I have gathered in my lifetime of cystitis experience.

I have this book to remind me of how to keep free of cystitis myself.

*I am the best proof that this stuff works and I'm passionate about helping you.*

If you follow *all* the protocols, then you should eventually be cystitis-free, forever. If used properly, this book may also change your life.

It's time to decide. You chose this book for a reason, and I know the solution you are looking for is inside. It may be one piece of information that you needed to hear, or it could be that most of it is new to you.

Please, don't be the person that holds the golden ticket and doesn't show up.

Don't wait until you have another bout of cystitis before reading this book and implementing the solutions to your problems.

Why not be the person who takes action now?

The advice in this book has proven to create positive long-lasting results: this is the solution you have been waiting for.

I'm calling you to action and holding out my hand. Shall we take this first step together to master your urinary health?

*I invite you on this fabulous road-trip. Coming?*

Take my hand, a deep breath, and let's launch this adventure.

I'll see you in the book.

# Chapter 1

# The Medical World of Cystitis

This is it! We begin our journey together. Excited? I am.

As you have seen in my disclaimer, I am not a medical doctor. I have a PhD in metaphysics that included natural health. This book is neither medical advice nor makes medical claims. It's based on my personal experience, my doctorate, and holistic certifications since the beginning of my metaphysical journey when I was 13.

As already mentioned, this is not a medical journal or a science-based research-paper, but it is worth mentioning that the medical world plays an important role in our journey and so here we explore why.

\* \* \*

The first cystitis that I can recall was when I was four, but I reckon I had it since birth, on and off. I was born with the cord around my neck and starving. I lacked in food and oxygen as nothing was getting through the umbilical cord. I was born six times, as I kept being pulled back up (poor mum!) and the doctor cut the cord off my neck from within: a blood bath.

I was so stressed, my heart was weakening and I was suffocating as the birth process was tightening my noose. I had to be resuscitated upon entry into the world.

I had no voice for four weeks. I made no sound at all as my larynx was so damaged. This resulted in a lot of throat issues throughout my life with huge repercussions metaphysically and socially, but that story doesn't belong in this bladder book.

I was a sickly baby and toddler. I was on antibiotics for infections regularly and I was on all sorts of medication.

Yes, the antibiotics may have saved my life, but the side-effect was it ruined my developing microbiome and so candida was rife from a young age.

That is what caused my chronic cystitis symptoms.

Antibiotics and dairy cause candida and kill off good gut flora: a double whammy. As I was starving, I went onto cow's milk formula very early. This was also not great for my development.

So, I started my life very dehydrated, starved, and with antibiotics and dairy. What made it much worse was adding sugar. Whilst being babysat by my grandmother for a week as my parents were working, one of her friends fed me lots of sugar. For days, the woman dipped my dummy into strawberry jam.

Jam is white sugar (glucose) and fructose (fruit). Every day, I had this 'treat', which apparently I loved. Of course, I would love sugar, it is highly addictive.

When my parents finally found out, they took me home straight away, and Dad took me to work with him, but the sugar had already caused its damage.

So, now add a ridiculous amount of sugar in an already damaged and struggling gut-flora, and my microbiome was truly set for candida. My weakened immunity and inflammation probably caused leaky gut and weakened all my systems and blood. This accounted for my low immunity, asthma, phlegm, eczema, poor sleep, strange hunger patterns, lots of crying, recurring infections and illnesses, and of course, my unknown cystitis symptoms.

I was a very needy baby and would only want to cuddle my parents. I would cry if anyone else wanted to hold me. I was a stroppy toddler, but I now know it was because I would have had cystitis most of the time.

As I said, at age four I knew I had it, I didn't know what it was called or that it didn't happen to everyone.

I was so used to feeling like shit that I thought that was how life was, and that everyone was struggling, so I didn't say much about it.

When it was really bad, then I would tell my mum that I had my funny tummy ache again and given digestive remedies, which clearly didn't help.

\* \* \*

Even as a young adult, I assumed all women had regular cystitis. I thought it was just what we had, like having periods.

\* \* \*

One day when I was off work again I told my mum I was on antibiotics for cystitis, and I flippantly said, 'well, it's been three weeks since my last one, so it's about right'.

Mum answered boldly that it was not right and that she only had cystitis *once* in her entire life.

This super-shocked me! So I started asking around, and it turned out that it wasn't 'normal', but as I had it all my life, I assumed it was.

I started on a mission to suss out 'why me' and what could I do about it. Not knowing that decades later, I would write a book to help others understand how to avoid it and that if anyone was suffering in silence, then I could be that voice that says:

*No! Cystitis is not part of being a woman, it's not normal, it should be talked about openly, & you can help yourself by following protocols.*

So, this is me shouting from a huge global rooftop in the centre of the Earth so everyone can hear, this book is my voice:

**'Cystitis is not a normal condition. It is not a taboo. It is not dirty. It is not shameful. And it can be avoided. You are not alone'.**

The cystitis type that I suffered mostly with as a baby and child was 'candida cystitis', and Overactive Bladder (OAB) with the occasional bacterial one (UTI), but I had so many antibiotics for my ENT issues (Ears Nose Throat) that I didn't get too many bladder infections, but rather chronic cystitis that you 'live' with. Well, no more.

**Candida cystitis is not acknowledged in the medical realm: it should be.**

I hope doctors will read this book and make candida cystitis common knowledge in the medical world so that they can help more people suffering from it.

How many times have patients complained of cystitis and yet there is no infection or blood present in their urine? Do doctors think we are making it up to get a sick-note? If there are no bacteria present, but the symptoms are there, it is obviously another *type* of cystitis, which is why I separated them into categories, more on that later.

The medical world can't help us with candida anyway, but they could inform patients of its existence and set them on a candida-starvation diet.

We need doctors for tests, medication, and when truly needed, surgery.

We can prevent cystitis ourselves reclaiming our power over our healthcare.

**Important Note**: I have to state that I am not against the medical world, they saved my life on many occasions and they sometimes do amazing work, but it depends on your doctor and urologist.

If I sound a bit off in this chapter, it is left-over residue from a certain few surgeons and doctors that were condescending and less than useful, to put it politely.

There are plenty of sympathetic doctors too. I have had a few kind and useful ones.

I'm giving a big hug and thanking the surgery/medical centre that I am with now. My current GP (a lady doctor in the UK) is amazing. Consultations with her are actually educational and she respects my natural ways and my need to know all my options and be in control of my health.

Doctors tend to class cystitis as an infection of the bladder, a UTI or Interstitial Cystitis (chronic) and not analysing or researching *why* it happens or giving any real precautionary measures, other than the advice of drinking more water and cranberry juice. I can't believe that is still what they recommend. Yes, to drinking more water, but in my past experience, they say that without asking how much we already drink.

When I was having 5 litres a day, a doctor told me to just have more water and cranberry juice and it will pass. I then said well how much water? He said oh, about 2 litres. When I explained that I was having *way* more, he was shocked.

My advice is to stay away from cranberry juice. Sugar in fruit is still sugar and all sugar cause inflammation and feeds candida.

Antibiotics will only work for a bacterial infection (UTI).

Antibiotics won't work for the other types of cystitis that I mention soon.

Antibiotics kill bacteria, they don't serve any other purpose.

The medical world can leave you deflated time after time as we put our trust in doctors to help combat a painful bladder, and they fail.

Sometimes doctors declare that no infection is present, and your heart sinks because you know you won't get antibiotics.

So you ask then, what is it that you do have because it feels like cystitis? And they don't know. A sympathetic doctor will sometimes offer you antibiotics just in case or if you have it often enough, will eventually refer you to a urologist.

If you are unlucky to have an unsympathetic doctor, as I did when I lived in London, you may be told to go home, drink more water, and get on with it. This may make you feel like a fraud, a hypochondriac and someone with low pain tolerance, and in reality, you are genuinely suffering.

These feelings can then lower your self-esteem and hope, adding to your already frustrated state and your anger intensifies, aiming at metaphysical cystitis issues.

**We explore the different types in the next chapter, so bear with me.**

Bladder candida, metaphysical, over-sensitive, or bladder IBS are not diagnosed by the medical world. There aren't any easy tests to prove their existence. They are diagnosed by your medical history, symptoms and trial and error.

**Medics do not acknowledge candida and metaphysical cystitis at all.**

I paid to see urologists several times, in different countries, when I was still not aware of why I was getting cystitis so often. And yes, when it was a bacterial infection, I was grateful to get the help, but it was my extensive research and my personal experiences that healed me once and for all.

I helped myself. Now, I'm helping you.

As a child, I would call my funny tummy, 'trouble', to myself. I would wake up in the morning and it would be there, and my heart would sink. I started my day saying to myself 'Oh no, I got trouble again today'.

The days that I woke up without it felt like Christmas.

I remember when I had 'trouble' I wanted to hide away from the world. I was irritable. I wanted to get away from it but I couldn't because it was inside me.

When I did ask for help nothing worked, so I gave up asking and lived with it.

This resulted in a frustrated child most of the time.

When I had 'trouble' during long car journeys, when my parents, sister and I would travel a lot, driving between England and France to visit family, it was hideous for me. I was stuck in a small space with people who irritated me, just because I was so uncomfortable and all I wanted to do was be alone in the dark and silence. I had to come up with some coping mechanisms.

So that I couldn't see my mum biting her nails, which *really* irritated me, I used to put my coat over my head, to make it dark. I still do this when I travel now, although not if I'm driving, obvs! It is a way to shut out the world, sometimes I would put my hands over my ears too as I was very sensitive to noise and I still am.

For me, noise intrusions are really irritating.

Perhaps it is because I had such poor vision since birth and no sense of taste for a while due to ENT issues, and so because of that my hearing is particularly sensitive?

Noise may not bother you such as nail-biting, slurping, noisy eating, or loud sneezing, but something else will. Whatever frustrates/irritates you chronically will have a personal link to your bladder. More on metaphysical links later.

I could hear my mum suck on fingers and crunch her nails and just the anticipation of it would make me tense. Frustration is linked to the bladder, so chronically being *pissed-off* means more chronic cystitis.

I came up with damage limitation strategies at a young age, as I had enough 'trouble' without having to put up with others irritating me, that I couldn't escape from, such as in a car, sharing a bedroom or being in a classroom.

I learnt, through trial and error, that taking deep continuous breaths and focusing on one thought or a happy memory helped, so in a way, I taught myself to meditate.

In frustration, I would also ask silently for help to anyone who would listen: God, the angels, the stars, the fairies, or my teddy bears. In a way, I taught myself to pray and be open metaphysically.

I would talk about 'trouble' and other problems with my imaginary friends. I liked them as they were fairies, floating spheres, or streaks of colours like the Borealis, or my bike that was really a black stallion or sometimes a unicorn.

I liked how it felt to be around them, much better than with most humans.

So, thinking back, it is no wonder that I was drawn to study metaphysics. It is no surprise that I become a cystitis expert, totally self-proclaimed, but well deserved.

I could be irritable but then bounce back so happy and want to cuddle people, play and smile. No, it wasn't bipolar or split personalities. It was cystitis or no cystitis.

I was unbearable when the pain and cramping were bad, or my wee burned, but when it would pass, I felt so much happier. I was no longer frustrated. I was so grateful. Oh, my, it was like Christmas and my birthday at once.

I would suddenly love life again, until the next bout when I recoiled from it and found any outside stimulus, especially people, most irritating.

So, due to my mood swings, I was called many nicknames, but one of them is 'Oh, the happy Jenny is back, and the sulky one is gone'.

I remember when I was a toddler my Nan asked me why I was so difficult and I shrugged 'I don't know, Nanny'. I guess the 'Bad Jenny' was led by cystitis, other ills or being too hungry, and the 'Happy Jenny' was led by feeling good.

Our bodies direct our lives, and our health and feeling good is so crucial to the quality of life and how we fit into our world.

*Can you relate to this? Have you noticed that your mood or the way you show up in the world changes when chronic health issues flare up?*

I could not blame it all on cystitis though, as other ailments wound me up too, one being my sight, resulting in me being so clumsy that I would annoy myself.

I had a constant painful throat, especially when I got angry, as my voice would cut out and my larynx got inflamed or infected, adding to my rage and not being able to speak up for myself when I wanted to.

I found so many injustices in the world and I wanted to fix them, seeing suffering or bullying made me angry and I wanted everyone to just get along.

There are countless factors that form our characters. The health of a child plays a vital role in how that child acts and sees the world and what belief patterns they form that will rule their life.

If I had 'trouble' at school I would play up and get told off, or sit in the toilet for ages. When I was at home or at my grandparents, I would take myself to my room, to be quiet, although as I shared a room with my sister, so if she was there I would go exploring elsewhere. Sometimes I would go outside, wherever, just to be alone.

Quiet, dark and by myself was the best place I could learn to tolerate my condition.

At this stage, I still thought it was normal to have this *trouble*. I did wonder how my sister just played and coped with this so well? The simple answer was she didn't have chronic cystitis.

From a young age, I learnt to tolerate pain and deal with frustration. When I was snappy, people would say I was an angry child. I had to apologise a lot, but in truth, I was just irritable because my bladder was, and people not understanding me just pissed me off.

When you are in chronic pain, it is very hard to be a part of the world properly.

As an adult, it's even worse, because you have responsibilities and you have to look after yourself, and others.

We can't very well sit at our desk or in a meeting with a coat on our head and hands over our ears, talking to fairies.

We can't say no to our children when they need feeding or caring for because we want to go to a dark room and hide under the duvet.

We can't tell everyone to 'fuck off' or to 'shut the fuck up' because we no longer just get sent to our room to think about it, as it now has proper repercussions.

As adults, we have less freedom to react how we want to, as there are too many social expectations, other people's rules, laws, and taboos that we are expected to abide by.

**So cystitis as an adult truly sucks too. It's never good, is it?**

So, throughout my life, I would go to the doctors, pee on a stick and confirm a bladder infection, get a course of antibiotics for UTI (urinary tract infection) ranging from three days to ten days. It would eventually go away and I would be grateful and happy to live again, until the next month when I went back for more medication.

I asked my GP why I kept getting cystitis and he said it was just bad luck.

**Note:** I don't believe in things *just happening.* Nothing is by chance.

*If we suffer from a condition there is a reason.* Just because the medics don't know why it doesn't mean it doesn't exist. There is a reason why you have bladder issues and hopefully, this book will lead you to the answers.

Once you know why you can deal with it.

Sometimes, I would pee on a stick and there was no infection, and I would explain that it feels the same, cramps, burning when I pee, irritable. And he would confirm he can't give me antibiotics, he looked up the urethra tube and swabbed it, and there was nothing there.

Sometimes there would be traces of blood or white bits in the urine but no infection.

Sometimes, there is no blood and no infection present, but the symptoms are still the same. For a simple organ, the things that can go wrong with a bladder are complex.

After so many times with cystitis, he finally referred me to a urologist, the first one I had seen. The waiting list was far too long, so I paid to go private, yes it was expensive, but as you know, when suffering from cystitis, we would pay anything to get rid of it.

I had an ultrasound over my full bladder, trying not to pee the bed. I then had an ultrasound over my empty bladder, to see if I had emptied it fully, and how it sits within the pelvic area.

My ultrasounds were fine, showing no problems.

We progressed onto an MRI to have a real good look. I was told I have a healthy bladder (well clearly I didn't).

We progressed onto an MRI with contrast/dye, to follow liquid going through the kidneys and into the bladder, to ensure no blockage or leaks anywhere in my urinary tract, but apparently, all was well.

We then progressed to a cystoscopy, a tiny camera and light on the end of a tube pushed up the urethra ( the pee tube) and into the bladder.

Had I not been awake, the specialist would have told me upon awakening that everything was fine, there was nothing to worry about.

*Luckily*, I had a throat infection at the time, so it meant no general anaesthetic, so I was awake during the procedure and saw for the first time inside my bladder and this had a profound effect on me.

There was no infection, he said the walls looked healthy, but as he turned the camera, half of my bladder walls were covered in white foam.

It looked like cotton wool or tall thin white mushrooms clumped closely together over some white surface.

I had already done some biology and candida research and it was obvious to me that something was not right, so asked if this white fluff was normal.

He replied 'it is just leucoplakia, some people have it, some don't, and it's nothing to worry about. There hasn't been much research as it's not worth it. It doesn't affect the bladder.'

I then asked if it was supposed to be there, knowing full well that it wasn't, but I couldn't very well be rude to him whilst he was inside my lady-bits.

He said no. I then asked, logically one would assume, seeing as nothing else is showing up on the tests, surely this white foam that is *not* supposed to be on my bladder wall *is* the cause of my cystitis issues?

He snorted, 'don't be stupid, I'm telling you: it's nothing.'

During the consultation afterwards, looking down at me from his glasses, he told me to go home, stop making a fuss, that there was nothing wrong with me, and he knew patients that were *truly* suffering from bladder issues, so I should stop wasting his time and to just live with it.

Yes, he actually said those words: Live.With.It.

Wow! I wondered how he would cope with his penis soaked in bleach, acid injected into his bladder and him squirming for decades, and then I charge him thousands of pounds to tell him to live with it? I shouldn't think he would cope anywhere as well as you and I have.

Twat.

What a colossal arse. And that is insulting arses.

## Linguistic Interlude

I'm aware that I use inappropriate swearwords that come out naturally and the above is a classic example. *Twat* and *bollocks* happen to be my go-to words as I love the way they feel in my mouth. When I pronounce them I mean, not the actual things!

By inappropriate I mean using body parts to denote anger or shame. Why use the word *Twat* as an insult? Vaginas are awesome and powerful and deserve more respect.

In the next chapter, I describe our vaginas and you will see that I call them *our precious holes*. These holes are often used as insults. What's the worst swear word? Most would say it's the *C-word*, which is another word for vagina, same as 'twat'.

Arse or butt swearwords also relate to that area.

Dick, prick, cock and bollocks swearwords relate to men's precious areas.

And 'fuck' is somehow now bad, but it originates as an abbreviation of 'For Unlawful Carnal Knowledge', which was the crime prostitutes were arrested for, so it wasn't a swear word or even a word but an abbreviation, but since someone decided to have sex outside marriage or getting paid for it is evil, it became a swearword.

So FUCK is a linguistic clue that somehow our society has adopted our private parts or a natural act (sex) to be rude, dirty, or bad.

So maybe we can invent new swearwords that don't insult any of our body parts.

So maybe instead of twat and arse, I could say:

'beeping beephead, beepsucking, limp-beeped motherbeeper' and let you choose the new words.

And maybe share them in our Facebook tribe (The Happy Bladder Tribe). The funnier, the better. Let's break this taboo of cussing. Swearwords are just words someone else decided were bad. The energy we put into them depends on our intention. If someone says 'I fucking love you, man' using 'fucking' as emphasis and not an insult, then it's not swearing. Just because someone somewhere decided a word was bad, it doesn't mean we have to agree or be bound by old traditions.

So, linguistic interlude over, back to the medical story…

\* \* \*

Sadly, I know I'm not the only one with similar encounters with specialists or doctors, NHS or private. I'm sure you have come across some too.

*What can you take away from it? How can you turn it into a positive?*

Actually, his attitude (Dr Beep-head) was exactly what I needed to spur me on to find my own answers and solutions, and so for that, I'm grateful that he sucked.

**It turned out I didn't need a specialist: I needed me.**

He had never suffered from cystitis and even when something was *so* obvious, he refused to acknowledge it and dismissed it. Ego issues anyone? God-complex?

This urologist was by far the most condescending doctor and has no business calling himself a urinary tract specialist.

He was unable to help me, and yet the answer was staring him in the face. It cost me a lot of money to be insulted. If I wanted that, I would have gone to the Monty Python Bureau.

*How much has cystitis cost you?*

Each 15-minute consultation with this so-called expert cost me £150, and that was going back almost 2 decades. The camera procedure alone was £2000. The ultrasounds and MRI's about the same. I have had 3 cystoscopies, several ultrasounds, and MRIs of my bladder over the decades in different countries. And I had plenty of NHS time and tests too for cystitis, which I don't know the cost as NHS is funded by UK taxes.

I have no idea how much my research has cost me, the countless hours of study, the blood tests, the antibiotics, the cystitis sachets, specialist foods, and of course, how much I had lost in earnings when I was so often unable to work.

**Financially, cystitis is a killer.**

*I so wished that this book existed when I was young.*

As I said, I got unlucky with my first urologist, but medical assistance is crucial in your bladder health to help rule stuff out.

You do need to have tests done if you are suffering to ensure there is nothing else wrong with the bladder, but do also keep this book, if you apply the protocols, it may save you so much in medical fees, useless medication, and will put you back in control of your bladder.

Do remember that doctors or GPs have studied basic medicine and so *basically* understand the urinary tract, but they haven't spent years solely exploring the bladder, and are not monitoring the latest research reports on it. They are general practitioners and know the basic stuff about the whole body and what medication to prescribe, they are trained in general medicine and pharmaceuticals. That is why they refer you to specialists for specific issues that they are unable to assist with.

A urologist specialises in the urinary tract. Urologists have studied further but only at the medical level. They *only* know about the physical bladder, not the whole body, nor the holistic bladder.

They don't take into account how the bladder is interconnected to all our body or emotions.

I don't consider them bladder experts. They are medically trained bladder specialists, and some are better than others. None of them will take the time or research to view your bladder holistically and be open-minded to consider metaphysical issues.

There used to be a taboo about candida in the general medical field, although now the microbiome area of medicine is coming to light, but for the most part, bladder candida is not acknowledged or studied, and any metaphysical issues are not even on the radar in medical terms.

The level of competence the doctors or urologists have will depend on their experience, how many people they have truly helped, the quality of their studies and their bedside manner. They are still not experts unless they have *experienced* for themselves what the condition they want to treat feels like and earned their dues by travelling through the painful journey and cured themselves of it.

An expert is someone with in-depth knowledge, personal experience and the wisdom to share the solutions effectively.

I felt the desperation when the medical world could not diagnose or help me. I was angry that I was made to feel like a whining little girl making up her pain, by a so-called specialist. The anger and frustration lead me to the best thing ever. It sent me on a rampage, fuelled by my hatred of the urologist's attitude.

**Back to the leucoplakia:**

I had already studied nutrition and candida in my previous diplomas, and so I recognised that the white foam looked like yeast, and the white wall it was on was leucoplakia.

I focused my research on candida in the bladder. There wasn't much at the time, given I didn't have the internet at home, and Google I don't think existed yet, so I couldn't ask him.

As with any experimentation, it came down to trial and error, using my findings to help myself and taking detailed notes. I had several journals on my bladder.

I discovered that candida can get into the bladder. Due to the bladder nature, it provides great conditions for candida to thrive, if you feed it well, but is not supposed to live there, and so it does cause irritation to the bladder lining, and it does interfere with normal bladder functions, and it does cause burning and cramps, just as leucoplakia does, no matter what that urologist said.

Anything that is not designed to be there will cause problems, that's logical, right?

I designed an anti-candida regime, which includes most of the protocols in this book and a very strict diet for 8 weeks to starve the candida and increase my good gut flora. By week eight, I was no longer suffering and I was on my way to recovery.

By starving the candida, I cured my chronic cystitis and IBS.

By adopting daily hygiene, sexual and toilet protocols, I stopped getting infections (UTIs).

By turning a negative into a positive, taking control of my health, and meditating into the related emotional issues, I cleared my metaphysical cystitis.

Eventually, I became cystitis-free. I was worried after month 1, fearing it would come back, then 3 months clear, then six months clear, that was unheard of, cystitis-free and completely symptom-free for half a year?

Never in my life had I had that, and I was in my thirties.

*Living without cystitis was revolutionary. Who knew life could feel so good?*

It was my own work that got me there, not the medics, although the medical tests helped to identify issues.

I had devised an emergency plan so that if I got a twinge, I would deal with it right away and it would settle. I was careful to engage all my protocols, but sometimes life happened, and I would push my luck and get a twinge, a warning signal.

So, my bladder-life was awesome, I was in the driver's seat and no more trips to the doctor, no more antibiotics, well, not for cystitis anyway.

The second time I had a camera in the bladder, it was much later, I had been cystitis-free for about seven years. I know right? Bladder Christmas every day.

So what happened? Well, I treated myself to a holiday in Spain to do yoga and meditation. I went alone, no big deal. I treated myself to a 4-star beach hotel. With a marble bathroom, clean with a bathtub, not just a shower cubicle. It was my birthday and I wanted a nice long hot bath. I hadn't suffered from cystitis for so long, I let my guard down: I didn't think about the water.

I knew not to drink it as most places in Spain, the water is not drinkable. Remember, if the water is not safe to drink, it is not safe to bathe in, but I had not come up with that protocol yet, as I never had cystitis from bad water, so it was not on my radar.

A shower probably would have been OK, but not soaking.

There was E-coli in the water. Later that night I did drink too much tequila with my new friend, but unknown to me, my bladder was already under attack. No countermeasures with that, I still would have ended up in the hospital because bathing in dirty water is never going to end well.

**Important note**: Think about it, your precious area, whilst submerged in hot water will relax and open up. Water will travel up all those holes, and microbes in the water will end up in your urethra and bladder, especially if like me, you bathe for hours as that is plenty of travel time.

Pay attention where you bathe. Even in your own bathtub where you trust the water, be careful what abrasive products you use to clean it, have you rinsed it properly? Do you use bubble bath or bath-bombs, if so: stop.

Things OK to use in bath water in my experience are Himalayan pink salt, Epsom salts, a few drops of organic essential oils that are well mixed in and not lemon or too acidic that could burn the skin, and seaweed. That's it, otherwise, just clean water.

At 4 am after my birthday bath and night out, I sat on the loo, cramped and burning. It was intensifying by the minute: cystitis.

Oh no, my heart sank. It was to be the worst case I had ever had, and I had stonkers.

Blood was no longer just coming out when I squeezed pee, but it was flowing out of my bladder continuously. My bathroom looked like a crime scene. I was too ill to ask for help. I couldn't leave the toilet and my lower body was numb from sitting on the loo seat too long. After what must have been a few hours, I transferred to the bath with hot water to try soothing the cramps, not realising yet that it was the water. Soon I was slumped in red, cold water. I climbed out and sat on the toilet again. The cramps were so bad that it felt like my bladder was going to give birth to itself.

I'm lucky that I didn't get bladder prolapse, and I'm *very* grateful for that.

I was short of breath and doubled up in agony.

When the emergency doctor finally got to me, she dipped the urine that I peed into a glass, it looked like Shiraz red wine. She could have just swabbed the bathroom.

She called for an ambulance right away. It was bad, I knew that.

I speak Spanish and so was able to tell the paramedics what happened, between heavy breathing and screaming, and holding my abdomen.

I was seen immediately in the emergency department at the hospital in Benidorm. I felt in safe hands. I was put on fluids right away and sent for a chest X-ray, which I found odd, but it was because my breathing was so laboured and painful. The chest was fine, it was a side-effect of being in so much agony, like being in labour, I'm told.

So yes, a bad cystitis infection can be life-threatening. As I said, cystitis *is* a big deal.

Luckily, the Spanish urologist did not tell me to 'live with it'. He got me on IV antibiotics, anti-cramp medication, painkillers, and plenty of IV fluids, and on the second day I was in theatre for a cystoscopy, and I was grateful for all of it as that time the medical world truly did save my life.

I looked at the screen during the camera in my bladder and I was pleased to see there was no candida, no leucoplakia. I knew, from my lack of candida symptoms that there hadn't been for several years, or if there was, it was slight and I was able to counteract it fast, getting rid of it before it could spread and take a good hold.

So it pleased me to see that.

However, I saw the scars on my walls, the urologist pointed them out to me, he said in Spanish, so I will paraphrase, 'ah, you poor girl, you have had many cystitis in your life, look your walls are so battle-scarred.'

I replied, 'yes, sadly, this is not my first cystitis-rodeo, Doctor.'

I amused him speaking Spanish even though I had a stranger up my bits, albeit a cute Spanish one with dark brown eyes and a dinky smile.

I heard my inner sarcastic voice, 'bloody typical, *now* you get close and personal with a gorgeous and kind Spaniard, I've only been waiting years. This isn't quite what I had in mind though, so next time, dating followed by foreplay and a proper bed, rather than numbing gel and stirrups with a stranger going straight to 3rd base, or whatever base urethra-penetration is. Deal?'

I smiled and answered myself in my head, 'No deal. No more sex, ever. No more anything. I want to curl up and die.' Cystitis had me once again and the 'Bad Jenny', was back.

I shut the voices up and continued focusing on the screen.

The scars looked like red pinkish spider webs on my bladder lining. I sent out a hug to my bladder in acknowledgement of all it had gone through since birth, and how it is still doing its best to be there for me. I felt humbled.

Then we saw it: the dreaded infection. He knew by then it was E-coli as the urine and blood results were back.

It looked like a bomb had it the wall, leaving a deep crater in it, a red angry bloody one with big broken veins pulsing, spewing out blood. It reminded me of a volcano erupting.

The E-coli had made a home, eating my bladder lining and it was still bleeding. I had been on two days antibiotics by then and so it had started to calm down. I can only imagine what it looked like when I was in the hotel bathroom. My poor bladder.

He kept me for 1 more day on IV and then told me to drink only 1 litre a day whilst I was on anti-cramping medication, as my bladder was so sensitive and overactive, it needed a rest.

This was the first time I heard this advice. I have to say the anti-cramping medication worked really well, and I did only drink 1 litre for two days only, as it didn't suit me and being in Spain, I was hot. I wanted to drink more, to flush out the germs and old blood. I also could only take the anti-cramping medication for a week as I suffered from side-effects of dry mouth and painful throat.

If it is an overactive bladder without infection or candida, then, yes, it could be a good idea to not drink much for a few days to allow it to rest and reset, but if there is an infection or candida, then the more fluid the better.

It's like pulling the chain on a dirty toilet: need to flush those germs out.

It took a week for the bleeding to stop. It got less and less as the infection went away. I was anaemic by then; the hospital was going to give me a blood transfusion but I refused. I said unless I fall in a coma, it is best not to have one, because it is a risk having a blood transfusion, they could get the wrong blood type which is a painful way to die, also there is a risk of further infection or blood rejection. I asked them to feed me and give me plenty of water and rest, and I will make up my own blood.

When I was discharged back to my hotel, I asked the urologist why I didn't have antibiotics to take back, only painkillers and anti-spasm pills. He said I had enough with the three days in IV. I insisted that in the past for bad infections in the bladder, I was given 10 days and this was worse, but he insisted, and so there was nothing I could do but trust the medical advice.

He was wrong.

As soon as the bleeding stopped and I was allowed, I flew home, with assistance and in a wheelchair, as I still was unable to walk much or carry bags.

A few days later I was rushed by ambulance to my local UK hospital.

As we waited for the ambulance that took two, yes 2 hours to turn up, my mum found me screaming on the sofa, it looked like I was convulsing. After the screaming, my lips were blue, my eyes pale and rolling around, I couldn't breathe properly and I was sweating, trembling with cold and my teeth were chattering.

I thought I was going to die. The UTI had seemingly gone, but I was not given enough antibiotics, and so the infection got into my blood and I got sepsis.

## Metaphysical Interlude:

A tribute to my little girl, *Tutz* (my cat that passed away a few months before, you can see her photo at the end of this book). We are going to explore more metaphysics later in the book, however, let this scene start that ball rolling…

When I could not breathe and it was looking really rather bad, I had a dying need (pun intended) to open my mobile phone. I had just enough control in my shaking arm to flip open the phone cover that was on the table next to me. Tutz was the photo background on my phone. She leapt out of the phone and onto my chest. As soon as she landed I took a deep breath and my breathing regulated. My lips slowly started turning from bright blue to pink, according to my Mum who witnessed the entire scene.

Once I was breathing again, and we could relax a little, Mum told me "Oh, my God, Jen, I saw Tutz fly out of your phone and jump onto your chest. It was like Professor McGonagall from Harry Potter when she turns into the cat and back again." I smiled and replied, "I know, Mum. I saw her too and she is still on my chest. My little girl saved my life."

We were humbled.

I knew I was going to be just fine, eventually. I had a vision of Tutz hissing at *Death*, the character from Monty Python and him mumbling as he disappeared.

The thing with these experiences is that some people will say it was just wishful thinking or a vivid imagination.

I say it really was Tutz from her after-death frequency helping me.

The thing is none of those theories can be proven. Those who say it is not real have no way of disproving it. So it comes down to what you want to believe, or rather what you just know is the truth.

\* \* \*

Once at the UK hospital, I got ample antibiotics, two very strong types, one for UTI and one for sepsis, and more fluids and painkillers.

Again, I was lucky that the medical world was there, it saved my life, although the sepsis was due to medical incompetence by not providing enough antibiotics for the original UTI in the first place.

I started making notes for this book on the back of an envelope which is all I could get hold of from my hospital bed. Mum then brought me a notebook and the outline for this bladder book was born. Two weeks later I was discharged, I was still anaemic and weak, but my bladder felt better. What a relief after seven days of bleeding in Spain and three weeks of constant cystitis, cramps and burning pee.

The last time I had a camera up the bladder was a month after sepsis in the UK, to make sure all was well.

This was a different experience than the last two. The anaesthetic they used was a gel that he inserted into my urethra and this was *horrid*. It gave me instant cystitis and urethritis so that burning feeling and inflammation of the urethra.

He said this was normal, I thought it nasty that they would use a numbing gel in the urethra and bladder that actually gives cystitis symptoms.

I came out of the examination room and cried, desperate not to have this feeling again. I drank lots of water and rested on my bed in the dark until it went away. It took about four hours, but I kept reminding myself that it wasn't real cystitis, but of course, it was, and so I came up with a new type of cystitis: medically induced.

The first urologist, yes, Mr Beephead, used an epidural to numb the area, somewhat overkill, but I didn't know any better as it was my first time. I may have had cystitis sensations after the procedure but the anaesthetic covered it up. I was a bit tender though once it wore off.

**The Spanish dude, by far my favourite, used an injection into my vulva to numb and that was fine, just a little prick, ah-ah, I'm used to those.**

I was sore and still had bacterial cystitis, so I didn't notice any medically induced cystitis then.

*When you have a cystoscopy, ask what type of anaesthetic or numbing cream they use and if possible, avoid the one that gives symptoms of cystitis or burning pee. If you need it, drink lots of water to flush the gel out as soon as possible.*

The UK NHS urologist, so my third camera, did not wait for the bladder to fill with the water and the gel before inserting the camera, because under NHS they are rushed as there are so many patients with bladder ills to get through. So, this haste enabled me to see a different side to my bladder, what it looks like when it is empty.

I didn't recognise it straight away, and then I understood. It was fascinating to watch, like a flower blossoming. At first, it looked like shrivelled intestine, twisted skin with lots of nooks and crannies as the skin was folded over itself. There was not much room as the walls were touching each other. Then, as the fluid was going in the tube, and the bladder was filling up, the walls grew apart and the twisted knots unfurled to become the wall lining. Soon I was looking inside a bloated balloon again.

I saw the two ureters openings and even witnessed pee coming into the bladder, it was fascinating. Not quite fascinating enough though to take my mind off the fact it was burning and the fear that my next pee would hurt.

The urologist assured me that it was only a sensation of cystitis and not true cystitis, but that is because the medical word classes the word cystitis to mean bladder bacterial infection because actually, I did have cystitis: an inflamed bladder and urethra irritated by the chemicals and the medical instruments.

I got to see inside my empty bladder, which provided a deeper understanding of why we get cystitis and how important it is to fully empty the bladder during a wee.

It's easy to see how germs, candida, or old pee get trapped in those folds. In the damp, dark, closed bladder, how they would be too comfortable and left to multiply. I noticed that the ureters were filling up the bladder with drops of pee, it takes a while for it to fill, but the more you drink, the quicker it fills up and so the less time it sits closed and trapping potential germs.

Hydration is key and I understood that at a deep level after my third camera, so for that, I'm grateful that he rushed to insert the camera.

**The first camera** procedure showed me what bladder-candida and leucoplakia look like, and the urologist's poor attitude pushed me on a rampage to get my own answers, so that turned out to be a real gift. He is still a Beep though.

**The second camera** procedure showed me what a bad infection in the bladder and scars look like. The urologist's attitude reminded me that just because they have medical diplomas, it doesn't mean they are right: I did need more antibiotics.

**The third camera** procedure showed me what an empty and unfurling bladder looks like, and how pee trickles in from the ureters. It also reinforced the importance of hydration. It flagged up a new type of cystitis too, the medically induced.

*What can you take away from any camera procedures in your bladder?*
*If you have not had one I suggest that you do, they can be illuminating.*

Writing this book is my last therapy on the subject, the penultimate piece of the puzzle. The very last piece is to set it free by publishing it hence sharing it with whomever it may help.

I was born with bladder issues, but I won't die from them.

I have healed myself. Now, it's your turn.

Do not wait until you have suffered for decades before having medical tests. I waited because I wasn't aware that cystitis wasn't normal and because, in the UK, you need a GP to approve you to see a specialist.

In some countries, you can pay to see whatever specialist without a doctor referral.

Consider getting all the tests done, to rule stuff out. It gives you the chance to see inside your bladder and this will help with creating a deeper connection. You can see for yourself if anything is wrong, rather than rely on the specialist's report.

I repeat, if you do have an infection, you need antibiotics. If it is a bad one, then go and get it checked afterwards to ensure all is gone. If you feel feverish, have trouble breathing, or are in pain after a UTI or any infection, please go to the hospital to be checked for sepsis as this condition is life-threatening.

Sepsis develops as a result of an infection somewhere that went untreated, or in my case, that was not treated for long enough.

The medics have a crucial place on your **Bladder A-Team** (we discuss the A-Team in Part Two) but do not rely on them for your bladder health, just rely on them for antibiotics when you need them, and for medical tests or surgery.

UK surgeries are so busy, that I'm sure GP's would be grateful for us taking control of our own health and start caring for our bodies better.

We can avoid many ailments and diseases by following the protocols in this book. The protocols will help with cystitis, with vaginal issues, IBS, food intolerances, inflammation in general, and so much more. More about that in Part Two.

## Chapter 1 Keynotes

- The medical world plays a vital part in our A-Team, more on that later.

- Cystitis and urinary issues are NOT normal or part of being a woman.

- It is important to have your bladder tested medically if you suffer from any cystitis or urinary issues.

- Do have antibiotics designed for UTI if you have bacterial infection cystitis.

- If after a UTI or any infection you feel feverish or in pain, check for sepsis.

- Urologists are not bladder experts if they have never experienced cystitis and not healed themselves.

- Most doctors or urologists are only medically trained and will help with physical bladder issues only, not metaphysical or candida.

- If your doctor or urologist is unsympathetic or insulting, you do have the right to find another one.

## Action! Interactive bit, it's your turn:

1. What experiences have you had with doctors or specialist about your bladder?

2. Have you been tested for a UTI and there was no infection, but there was blood or white bits detected in your urine? This is a

sign of another type of cystitis. We delve into those soon, but just make a note of times you suffered from a bladder or urinary issue.

3. Have you had a camera in your bladder? Can you learn anything from it?

4. If you have not had your bladder tested, contact your doctor now and ask for tests, go private if you have to. Use the medical facilities to help diagnose your bladder problems, or in most cases, rule stuff out.

5. Get a large notebook to use as your journal during our journey together. Use it to answer the interactive questions at the end of each chapter and note anything that comes up for you.

For convenience, I will be publishing a workbook for notetaking called *'Piss to Bliss Companion'*, but you can use a blank notebook if you prefer.

So, we have explored how the medical world can help with cystitis. We know that my experiences with medical tests helped me come up with my own solutions. So, it's time to get to know *exactly* what cystitis is and what I mean by different types.

I chose to put my medical history chapter first so that you get to know me better straight away as it involved quite a few personal stories, and hopefully, you have made notes about yours, maybe even shared some in our Facebook group.

So, as now we are well acquainted and besties, it's time to get technical, so let's get straight into chapter 2.

## CHAPTER 2

# 25 Different Types of Cystitis

I have written this book in a relaxed tone to share information in a digestible way, not condescending, confusing or fear-mongering. Remember, this book is a self-help guide, it is not a medical journal, even though this chapter looks quite technical.

My vision is that it also brings hope, comfort and a sense that you are not alone in your suffering. So, hand-in-hand, here we go. Ready?

\* \* \*

**What are the origins of the word *cystitis*?**

Cystitis means inflamed bladder. The word *cyst* or *cystis* means bladder or bag.

Adding '*-itis*' to the end of a word originally showed possession (I belong to the noun), but now it depicts 'inflammation'. If you put it after a noun it describes inflammation/swelling of that thing. Sinusitis is an inflammation of the sinuses, arthritis (arthr is ancient Greek for joints) is an inflammation of the joints, laryngitis is an inflammation of the larynx (voice box), and so the list goes on.

So, all cystitis *really* means, is an inflammation of the bladder.

\* \* \*

Separating cystitis into types (or causes) helped me to see the bigger picture. Pieces of a puzzle that brought me to create the 'protocols', more on those in Part Two.

The cystitis types (so the main reason why the bladder is inflamed) that are most well-known and mostly treated by the medics tend to be these three:

- Urinary Tract Infection (UTI)
- Interstitial Cystitis (IC) also known as Bladder Pain Syndrome (BPS)
- Bladder Cancer

I have had the top two, however, the medical solutions didn't always work, which lead me to believe those three types were only the tip of the iceberg. I went digging to find out why I kept getting bladder problems and that is how I came up with the following 25 types.

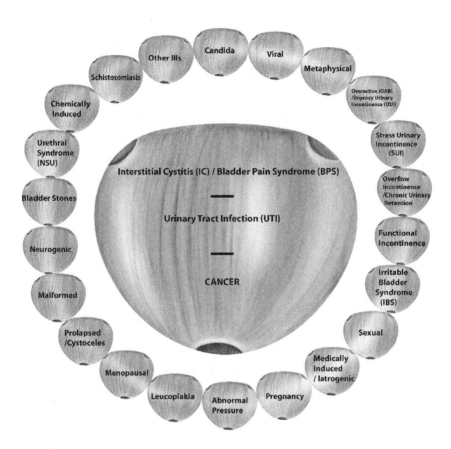

© Dr Jennifer Meyer

Not all types are official categories in the medical world and others may not class these as *cystitis* but I do because all these causes can irritate the bladder in some way, and remember cystitis just means inflammation of the bladder, so knowing these issues that potentially affect the bladder was crucial in my learning.

**See the illustration above that I designed**: the large bladder shows the three most known bladder problems (causing a type of cystitis) and on the peripheral, 22 mini bladders each with their own reason to cause a type of cystitis, but that are less known and some not known to the medical world.

The solutions to help all types are similar, but I find it crucial to understand the nitty-gritty, as sometimes our missing nugget of gold lives in the details.

This is your own private treasure hunt, so what piece of information in this book will help you connect the dots to the knowledge you already have to solve your bladder issues? I'd love to know.

*Bear with me, this chapter can get a tad technical. For now, we only touch on the types, as we delve deeper into them later.*
*As you read through the possible types of cystitis, put a tick next to the ones that you recognise or are aware that you may have suffered from.*

### In my opinion, there are 25 reasons for/types of cystitis:

### 1- Interstitial Cystitis (IC)/Bladder Pain Syndrome (BPS)

This is a condition causing an inflammation of the bladder lining creating pain and pressure. Interstitial suggests that the inflammation is also in between layers of tissue, so not just the top layer of the bladder walls. In some people, it comes and goes but in others, it is a constant companion, which is why I class this type, as well as the 'candida cystitis', as chronic cystitis.

IC is not caused by an infection rather a chronic condition that resembles autoimmune problems.

The pain increases as the bladder fills up, especially in those with smaller bladders. This pain can also spread to the whole pelvic area. There is a need to pee frequently during the day and night, leading at times to urgency: an urge that doesn't go away, even after a wee.

Unfortunately, this is a common bladder complaint especially in women, and some men diagnosed with 'prostatitis', may have undiagnosed chronic cystitis.

**Bladder ulcers** also called 'Hunner's lesions or patches', are part of IC and are not the same ulcers that you get elsewhere. They are specific patches of inflammation on the bladder wall related to IC.

## 2- Bacterial Infection Cystitis/Urinary Tract Infection (UTI)

This is one of the most common and is the only one where you will need antibiotics.

This cystitis is caused by bacteria that have entered the bladder and attacked the lining. This type has a limited life-span as the bacteria will eventually die off, and much faster and more effectively with the right antibiotics and it is the easiest to diagnose. A UTI is a bacterial infection anywhere in your urinary tract, so the kidneys, ureters, bladder, sphincter or urethra. It is possible to have an infection in your kidneys and bladder at the same time, or just in one place.

### 3- Candida Cystitis

This is not an infection but an infestation of candida, yeast, bad gut bacteria or thrush, inside of the bladder. This is common, even though not talked about or acknowledged in the medical world. This is not helped by antibiotics or cranberry juice but worsened by them, as all sugars, including fruit, feed the candida. I call this chronic cystitis. Cystitis will last as long as the overgrowth of candida in your bladder does. These yeasts can live forever if not dealt with.

I class this as chronic cystitis and sufferers of this, like IC once they have got rid of it will learn to live carefully so not to get it again, or rather so it does not flare up.

### 4- Viral Infection Cystitis/Epstein-Barr Virus (EBV)

Like when you have the flu or a common cold, it is viral and so antibiotics do not affect it. Luckily, these viruses do have a limited lifespan and will die off eventually. The exception is EBV that can hang around for years or a lifetime, sometimes undetected. It can mimic symptoms of many ailments such as thyroid problems, lack of energy, autoimmune and urinary issues. If you have had glandular fever anytime in your life, then chances are you also got this. EBV can be identified by a blood test.

### 5- Metaphysical Cystitis

This type is not acknowledged in the medical world. The source is not physical but rather emotional, mental, or spiritual and has rippled-effect, affecting the physical bladder, but may be called as an unknown origin or unexplained cystitis or pelvic pain. This doesn't show up on medical scans or tests, but it is still very real. To deal with this type, we need to uncover the original point of impact and deal with that.

### 6- Overactive Bladder (OAB)/Urgency Urinary Incontinence (UUI)

Uncontrollable bladder spasms and pain resulting in the urgent need to pee and potentially wetting yourself frequently. There seems to be no warning or ability to hold on. The medics do not class this as a disease but rather a chronic condition.

### 7- Stress Urinary Incontinence (SUI)

This is where the urethra (pee tube) can no longer take the pressure of urine from the bladder and so it leaks. There isn't a proper closure at the sphincter. You can pee just a few drops or leak an entire pee. It is called *stress*, as in pressure, so it comes on mainly with activities such as sneezing, laughing, coughing, lifting or exercising. It is possible to get both bladder (UUI) and urethra (SUI/Overflow) incontinence at the same time and this is classed as **Mixed Incontinence.**

### 8- Overflow Incontinence/Chronic Urinary Retention

Overflow incontinence is often caused by a blockage or obstruction in your bladder, sphincter or urethra, and so the urine pushing behind the blockages finds a way around and leaks out.

It is also when your bladder doesn't give the signal to pee even though it is full, and so wee leaks out as it has no choice, the full bladder pushes the wee uncontrollably.

### 9- Functional Incontinence

This is where the person is aware of the need to pee but doesn't go. There could be physical reasons such as there is no toilet available or they are disabled in some way and do not have a catheter.

It can also be an emotional or mental issue that stops them urinating such as confusion, dementia, depression or anxiety, fear of the dark, being bullied, or refuses to use the toilet in public or in front of others.

This is also when someone pees themselves through fear.

I class **Bedwetting** in this type too.

If they hang on too long, they are likely to wet themselves and empty their bladder involuntarily and this is why it is classed as incontinence.

## 10- Food Intolerance Cystitis/Irritable Bladder Syndrome (IBS)

What causes irritable bowel syndrome can also irritate the bladder.

This cystitis is inflammation caused by certain foods, drinks, stress, and an unhealthy lifestyle.

## 11- Sexual Cystitis

This is an irritation or inflammation of the bladder, urethra, vagina, or anus, yes anus, due to sexual intercourse trauma. Any sex will leave that area vulnerable, even soft love-making, but this type should settle down. Yet, it can evolve to other types of cystitis if bacteria, viruses, foreign bodies, or sexual abuse occurred during sex. To be clear though, cystitis is not a sexually transmitted disease. Much more clarification on this later! This type is also known as *honeymoon cystitis*.

## 12- Medically Induced Cystitis/Iatrogenic

This is a direct result of medical intervention such as surgery on the bladder/kidneys or urethra; the effect caused by the dye in MRI contrasting for urology; the numbing gel inserted into the urethra and bladder for a cystoscopy (a camera in the bladder). This gel gives an instant feeling of burning, which is an irritable symptom of cystitis. It does go away after drinking plenty of water to flush it out, but it can last up to 24 hours. The use of catheters, a tube inserted in the urethra into the bladder, will most likely also cause cystitis. Although medically necessary, there are things do to avoid cystitis from such procedures and we go into that later.

## 13- Pregnancy

Cystitis can be common during pregnancy. As the baby grows the womb expands and taking up more than its usual share of the pelvic area, hence pushing on the bladder or the bowels. This pressure will obviously irritate it and make you want to pee more often and more urgently.

The hormone fluctuations may also affect your bladder as well as all of your systems.

## 14- Abnormal Pressure Cystitis

Any lump in the pelvic area may aggravate the bladder.

So any cysts, fibroids, stones, lumps or cancer, growing *anywhere* in the pelvic area, could be pushing against the bladder, creating cystitis and incontinence symptoms.

## 15- Leucoplakia Cystitis

Leucoplakia is a mucosal disease showing up as white patches and lesions on the bladder walls. Medical science has not really done too much research on this and leucoplakia in the urinary tract is considered rare. However, *rare,* I had it, so don't let rarity put you off getting checked for this if you have symptoms.

A camera in the bladder and possible biopsies of the tissue will identify it. Medically there doesn't seem to be any treatment, although this can be a premalignant condition, so it is advised to have it diagnosed and followed up regularly.

The symptoms are typical cystitis: painful pee, an uncomfortable pelvic area, urge to pee frequently, difficulty peeing, blood in urine, sometimes white bits in the urine.

I found that treating my candida cystitis also got rid of leucoplakia, eventually.

## 16- Menopause Cystitis

Once we start menopause we release less and less oestrogen. This can dry the vaginal area and the skin inside the urethra, giving a sense of cystitis and discomfort whilst peeing and even when not. It can cause urethritis.

Hormone fluctuations and issues can also play a direct part in bladder problems, as well as in other systems.

## 17- Bladder Cancer

Like anywhere in the body, cancer cells can be in the bladder. As in all cancers, the progress is rated in different stages. It can be the primary meaning cancer started in the bladder or secondary, it started elsewhere and migrated there.

Sometimes kidney cancer can result in bladder cancer. Urinary cancer can be anywhere in the urinary tract, in multiple areas, or just in one place, such as the bladder.

## 18- Prolapsed Bladder/Cystoceles/Fallen Bladder

This is a mechanical issue, not necessarily an internal bladder problem.

If the vagina wall gets weak, then it gives way and can no longer fully supports the bladder. When this happens, the bladder dislodges itself and it sinks.

The level at which it has dropped is differentiated in classes, there are 4 stages of prolapse and we detail these in a later chapter.

## 19- Malformed Bladder

This is a mechanical issue where the bladder or urinary tract system defected during formation in the womb.

Usually, malformation of the bladder means there are likely to be other formation issues, such as spina bifida.

If, as a baby, you had surgery for a defected urinary tract, then it may have left that area weak and prone to cystitis.

## 20- Neurogenic Bladder

This is a specific issue due to a nerve problem, either temporary or permanent.

It could be temporary, such as damaged coccyx and the inflammation pinches the nerves related to the bladder and urethra.

It can be permanent if you damage the spinal column anywhere.

Damaged or severed nerves are very problematic.

This is an issue with the nerve signals to the bladder or within the bladder.

## 21- Bladder Stones

These are balls of minerals and calcium that form in the bladder. They can vary greatly in size and either small enough to pee out, or they get too big and may cause blockages and cystitis.

## 22- Urethral Syndrome/Symptomatic Abacterriuria/ Non-Specific Urethritis (NSU). Urethral Stenosis/Stricture

This is an irritated, inflamed or narrowed/restricted urethra. It is possible to have this condition without having problems in the bladder. Sometimes when you just feel burning whilst and after peeing and discomfort in that area but no pain or spasms in the bladder or no frequent need to pee, it could be just the urethra that is problematic. I still class this as a type of cystitis as the urethra is linked to the bladder, and if it is an infection it could infect the bladder. Most cystitis will also cause pain in the urethra. This could be caused by an infection, dirty sex, food intolerance, basically the same reasons as bladder cystitis.

If medics don't find a reason for urethra problems then it is classed as non-specific.

## 23- Chemically Induced Cystitis

Exposure to certain chemicals in some industries can cause urinary issues.

Chemicals in cigarettes are also linked to urinary problems.

Exposure to daily chemicals found in most commercial daily cleaning and beauty products can also irritate some people and be linked to cystitis.

## 24- Schistosomiasis/Snail Fever/Bilharzia

A disease caused by flatworm parasites that infect the urinary system and intestines. This is mainly caught by drinking or swimming in infected water.

## 25- Other Ills Linked to Cystitis or Vaginal Area

There are other problems not located inside the bladder that could cause symptoms of cystitis, or affect your vaginal area, such as a damaged coccyx, diabetes, lichen, fibromyalgia, dementia, chronic fatigue, bacterial vaginosis, vaginal dryness, female genitalia mutilation, sexually transmitted diseases. In addition, for men, also prostate and scrotum issues.

I have grouped them together as *type 25 cystitis* and go into detail in chapter 4.

* * *

Separating the types of cystitis in this way helped me to understand why sometimes antibiotics helped, and sometimes not, because the symptoms of each type are similar but the cause is different, and so the medical solutions differ, but as I mentioned, it is common for doctors to class most cystitis under 'bacterial infection', or 'UTI' urinary tract infection, but most of the time, it isn't.

**This finally sheds light on why we keep getting cystitis: because we don't keep getting the same type.**

Medical solutions such as antibiotics, other drugs, and cranberry juice may help one, but encourage another type, such as candida, and so the suffering continues, without much relief between bouts of bladder trouble.

Doctors and urologists, in my experience, only recognise some types of cystitis and the solutions they offer are antibiotics, drinking more water, taking sachets, and drinking cranberry juice, and eventually offer pessaries, questionable medication, operations, or removing the bladder in extreme cases.

Antibiotics may only work for bacterial infections. Cranberry juice or antibiotics for other types could aggravate the bladder further, contributing to a weakened state and recurring cystitis of different types.

**Note**: to confirm if you have a bacterial infection, a doctor will test your urine. They dip it immediately and confirm if blood and/or bacteria are present, they may need to send it off to the lab to grow cultures to identify the exact type of bacteria, as this may affect which antibiotic they prescribe, but there are UTI general antibiotics that should be enough, at least until the results are in.

It is very important that you go to the doctors if you have any cystitis, to confirm if there is an infection and to get the proper treatment. Please do have the antibiotics if they will help, if you don't, your bladder may not be able to cope and the infection could leak into your blood and you go septic.

Tests to identify infection in the urine are not always accurate and don't always pick up an infection, even if there is one. It is, however, the best option we have at this stage. Sometimes infection does show up, so it is still worth going to be checked out when you have any form of cystitis. Ask what bacteria is present and which antibiotics are targeted for that specific bug and start being an active part of your treatment when you seek medical help: take your power back.

**Don't assume the medically qualified are experts on bladders, especially not yours.**

## Chapter 2 Keynotes

- There are 25 types of/reasons for cystitis.

- The gold is in the details, what treasures will you find?

- Medical practices are not always effective at solving cystitis or bladder issues properly or permanently.

- If you have genuine bacterial infection cystitis (UTI), you need appropriate antibiotics and for the proper length of treatment.

- Medication, antibiotics, cranberry juice will not help most types of cystitis.

- Doctors and medical specialists are not always genuine bladder experts.

- Implementing the protocols in this book (coming up later) should improve all of your health, not just the bladder.

## Action! Interactive bit, it's your turn:

1. What have you read in this chapter that has surprised you?

2. How many types of cystitis do you think you have experienced in your life?

3. Have you ever been to the doctors for cystitis and they were not able to help?

So, we have identified the 25 different types of cystitis and later we will explore how to avoid getting them, but for now, let's discover what the bladder does.

What are our *Waterworks*?

Let's find out. We are arriving in chapter three.

# CHAPTER 3

# Bladder Function/About Our Waterworks

What is the bladder about? What do our waterworks do? What is our urinary tract?

I have designed my own illustrations to help clarify, as my Pop said a picture paints 1000 words.

I ask you to look at your vulva (what I lovingly call your flaps) now, get naked and use a hand-held mirror or look in a large mirror and explore. There is nothing wrong with that. Get to know your body fully.

## Female Anatomy

I will call your lady-bits, so your vagina area: *your precious holes.*

Women have a clitoris (part of the female sexual pleasuring gland) that sits hidden sometimes (blanketed by your flaps) at the top of your vulva.

We then have 3 precious holes in the vulva area:

1. The top one is our urethra, a hole leading to the tube that connects up to our bladder, part our urinary tract system. Where we pee from.

2. The middle hole is our vagina, a tunnel leading up to our womb, a part of our reproductive system, where we menstruate or give birth from.

3. The last hole is our anus, opening to our rectum, colon and intestines, a part of our digestive system, where we poo from.

Please see all the illustrations. Familiarise yourself with the pelvic area inside & out.

## Male Anatomy

**Men have 2 precious holes in their area:**

1. The hole at the tip of their penis also called a urethra, which leads to their bladder and their testes. Through this hole, they pass urine and semen, although not at the same time. Men's urethras are, by design, much longer than in women, as it runs through the penis before entering their body cavity and then the bladder. This is one reason why men usually get fewer UTIs than women. Men do suffer from bladder issues too.

2. A hole called the anus leading up to the rectum, colon and intestines. This hole is the same as in women. For the most part, the men's two holes are very far apart and never the twain shall meet, limiting the risk of transferring faecal matter or germs from one hole to the other.

**The following 3 illustrations show us:**

1- **Our waterworks, so how the kidneys and bladder connect.**

2- **Our flaps and precious holes**

3- **Our female pelvic area on the inside**

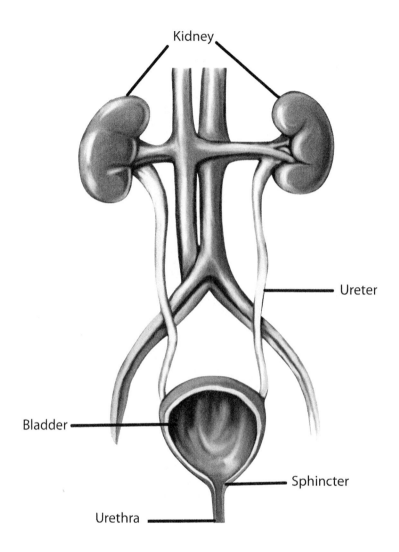

Copyright Dr Jennifer Meyer

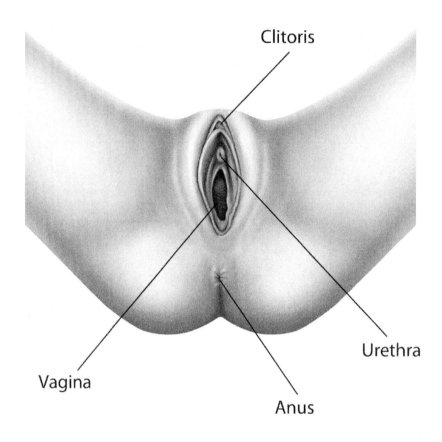

Copyright Dr Jennifer Meyer

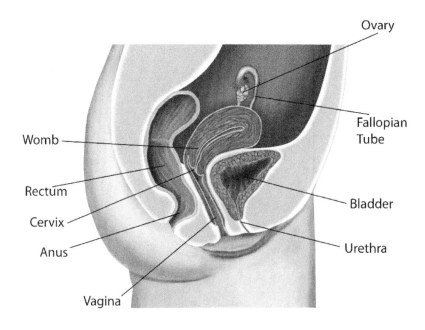

Ovary

Fallopian Tube

Womb

Rectum

Cervix

Anus

Vagina

Bladder

Urethra

All women have three holes but not all are the same dimensions.

In some women, the distance between these holes is closer.

In some women, the urethra is shorter or narrower, and although medically similar, all women's vaginas are different too, just as men's penises are not identical.

All bladder capacities differ also.

This is an important fact to consider as women with closer holes, shorter urethras, and smaller bladders are more prone to getting cystitis.

**Our Waterworks/Needing A Wee**

The bladder is a part of our digestive system called our urinary tract. What we drink and eat is filtered by the liver. The large waste is then passed into the intestines (to make poo) and the small particles go into the blood, which is then filtered by the kidneys. The kidneys clear out toxins, excess salts, water and minerals and locks them into the water to make urine.

The kidneys then send this urine down the ureters, the tubes attaching the kidney to the bladder. We have two kidneys. Each kidney has its own ureter leading into each side of the bladder.

Once the bladder reaches near full capacity, the pressure pushes on the nerve endings in the walls telling our brain that we need to pee. The pressure then pushes on the sphincter, the muscle-plug at the bottom of the bladder, which opens to the urethra and out. We then get in position, relax and allow the sphincter to spiral open, at this point the bladder walls, sphincter and urethra muscles will contract to push the urine down the tube, exiting the body.

Once the flow stops, the sphincter closes and the bladder shrinks to its empty state.

If all parts of that system are healthy, so kidneys, ureters, bladder, sphincter, urethra and all nerve endings, and spinal nerve channels, then this process is painless.

The kidneys do the cleaning up and create urine. The bladder's job is to store it and then pass it out of the body, ready to receive fresh wee.

It is a holding station, without it, we would be continuously peeing.

When empty, the bladder looks like a small twisted piece of intestine. As it fills up, it untwists and opens out, and when stretched, it's a round smooth ball. The lining is flesh coloured. It is a bag with three openings. At the top, there is one on each side, opening to the ureter going to each kidney, this is designed as a one-way valve so only urine coming from the kidneys can pass down, not urine from the bladder back up to kidneys if all goes well. There is one opening at the bottom to let out the urine.

**:o) A Happy Bladder Function:**

That's it, our waterworks are a simple design and if treated well, does a quiet job.

Yet so many factors can upset the system, and here we focus on the bladder. Luckily, knowledge is key, and once we know how to avoid upsetting it, it will be a much easier ride to happy bladder health.

A happy bladder should not be felt until about ¾ full of urine, and then we get the signal to pee, that slight sensation of heaviness and the desire to release, but no pain or discomfort. At this point, we should be able to hold on and continue to a full bladder, although it is best to pass urine as soon as we feel we need to.

We have strong muscles in the bladder and surrounding it in the pelvic floor area, and we can usually squeeze these muscles hard, holding our bladder tightly and supporting it as it becomes heavier with urine and pushing down on our vaginal wall. Then we squat and relax, giving our brain the signal that we are ready to release and the sphincter in the bladder can go ahead and open, and our muscles can push, and then we pee.

Peeing should be painless and rather enjoyable as we get relief from the pressure when the bag empties. We should not feel happy kidneys either, at all. The only part of our waterworks we should feel is the bladder when almost full, that's it.

### :o( A Sad Bladder Function:

A sad bladder may communicate in various ways: a dull ache in that area; a sharp pain; an irritable sensation that you can't get away from; anger; frustration; spasms and cramps; blood in the urine; burning sensation as you pass wee; a stabbing or electrifying nerve pain from your urethra, shooting up the tube into the bladder; an involuntary squeezing; fever; shortness of breath through long periods of pain and exhaustion; depression and despair. These are all great reasons to do what it takes to keep your bladder a happy one, right?

Kidneys will also let you know in a painful way if there is a problem. It could feel like you have been punched in the lower back, both sides or just one side; be really sore; sometimes doubled up in pain; swollen; feeling sick; vomiting; fever, and blood in the urine.

You can have just a kidney infection without it affecting your bladder and urethra or, most likely, Pyelonephritis, when a bladder infection has also spread up to the kidneys.

It is also possible to have cystitis or UTI in the bladder, without it affecting the kidneys.

## Why Cystitis Happens

So, let us understand why our bladders get sad and what we can do to fix that.

It's time to take control of our health.

It does not reside in the medical world, society, or taboos.

It's our body, our bladder, our choice and our responsibility.

## Responsibility doesn't only mean being in charge but also able to respond.

**Note:** I will repeat myself quite a bit in this book and this is on purpose. Repetition helps the information sink in deeper. We are on a new journey, an extensive one and it's important to take our time to let it all sink in.

Agreed? Brill.

Everything we eat, drink, inhale or touch will be in our blood and eventually connect with our bladder. Whatever goes in one end of the digestive tract (the mouth), will go through it all, ending up at the other end, so either the anus or the urethra.

This is great news, as it means we can now take control of what we allow through our tract. We decide what will go in the urine and what will, therefore, sit impregnating our bladder walls. The fewer toxins and inflammatory foods and drinks we consume, the less will be in our pee and therefore less will be touching our bladder wall.

**Catheter**

There are three types of catheters.

1. An indwelling, for permanent use and it is lives inside the bladder
2. A temporary/intermittent catheter, inserted in the urethra for a short time
3. External catheter like a huge condom placed over the penis to capture pee

Here I talk about the temporary one as it is the most common.

This is a plastic tube that is inserted inside the urethra then through the sphincter and into the bladder. There are several reasons why you may need a catheter at times. A temporary one may be used if you have mobility issues and are unable to walk to the toilet. This could be as a result of an operation, broken limbs, or short-term nerve damage and it will eventually be removed.

Catheters can also be for long term use for people in comas or with permanent spine or nerve damage, which either stops them using their legs or disrupts the nerve signals to the bladder.

In the short term, catheters are not too problematic as long as inserted, removed, and monitored correctly. They are, however, a possible source of infection for they create a permanent opening from the outside straight into the bladder, because the sphincter is wedged open so that pee can flow out continuously.

This affects, as in weakens the muscles of the bladder as with any muscles if you don't use it, you lose it. It is also a foreign body inside the bladder and urethra and your body may, quite rightly, take offence and try to eject it, the same way a womb sometimes reacts to a coil being inserted in its opening.

If catheters are needed, I offer a few tips on keeping it friendly for your bladder.

**Catheterisation Tips:**

1- Ask for your pee (that ends up in a bag) to be dipped frequently to ensure there are no infections or blood, as sometimes a UTI cannot be felt as much because pee is forced out.

2- Ensure the area is clean, if unable to wash, ask your nurse or carer to make sure, when going for a poo that all faeces is properly removed, the whole tube and bag of the catheter is sterile, and anyone touching it uses clinical gloves and antibacterial products.

3- Ensure the bag is emptied before it is full to avoid blockages so the bladder can continue emptying effortlessly at all times.

4- Keep an eye on the colour of the pee, it should be clear to slightly yellow and no darker than straw colour. If it looks too dark, like orange squash, brown, or red, there is a problem, it could be anything from slight dehydration to an infection or, in the worst-case scenario, cancer.

5- Do the bladder meditation to create a healthy flow of connection and then you can explain to it why it has been invaded by a foreign tube and how to best work with it. This may sound bonkers to you, especially if you are medical or not at all woo-

woo, but go with it, what have you got to lose? (See meditation chapter).

6- Only trained people should insert and remove catheters, not just anybody. It may pinch as it goes in and comes out, but other than that, you should not be in pain. It may feel uncomfortable at first, as your urethra is not used to being continuously stretched, but find a way to be OK with it, as resistance will not help. That is the same for anything. Pun intended: go with the flow…

7- Consider a weekly bladder wash to ensure the whole tube and the bladder is cleaned and totally unblocked. This needs to be done by a trained medical professional.

8- Ensure you are fitted with the right size catheter as they come in different diameters.

Long term use of catheters can be problematic causing infections, discomfort and of course, loss of bladder contraction functions.

At times it is necessary, so it is what I call, '**damage limitation**', and still do the best we can for our bladder under whatever circumstance we find ourselves. There is always something we can do to help ourselves, no matter how small as it all counts.

Please don't despair, and remember to let out any frustration or anger, you have every right to be pissed off. The idea is to allow emotions out and not to hold them in. Anything you hold onto, hold in, refuse to let go, or fight against the flow, is energetically stored in your bladder. It's time to get rid of those trapped emotions and free yourself. Your bladder will be grateful.

I will help you with the energy bladder part later in the book. I'm just sowing the seed so when we get to the juicy metaphysical bit of our journey, it will already be familiar.

* * *

If you have cystitis of any kind your body will communicate this to you in various ways. You may only have one or two symptoms, or the whole package, depending on the severity of the swelling and the type/cause of it.

**Extensive List of Potential Symptoms of Cystitis or Other Bladder Problems. Remember you may experience only one or two of these and each bout of cystitis may be different. Cystitis does not specifically mean a UTI, it can mean ANY type of cystitis:**

- Dull ache in your lower belly or lower back

- Gripping pain in your pelvic area or lower back

- Being thirsty, dehydration symptoms

- Dry vulva or urethra skin

- Pain and discomfort in your bladder area

- A heavy sensation on your pelvic floor

- A burning when you pee as if it were acid

- Always needing to go to the toilet, but there is nothing there

- Incontinence

- Frequent or an urgent need to pee

- Blood in the urine

- Blood coming from the bladder even when not peeing

- Uncontrollable squeezing of your urethra, especially after peeing, even after a 'fake pee', when there is nothing there

- Sharp pain up the urethra, like having a blow-dart shot up there, or being stabbed

- Electricity surging up your urethra like a dentist drilling a tooth and hitting a nerve

- Laboured breathing

- Swelling, inflammation of the abdomen and the vulva

- Exhaustion

- Confusion

- Sadness, crying, irritation

- Depression

- Anger, being pissed off

- Aggravated by piss-takers

- Frustration

- Despair

- Passing out

- Fever

* * *

## Linguistic Interlude and Clues

I'm a linguist and love to study words. Our ancestors left us clues when inventing language, reflecting how we used to be more aware of our bodies. The words may have changed with time, but the meanings remain. We were great storytellers.

**Notice how we use phrases related to the bladder or urine to denote negative emotion:**

- *Pissed off.* Means you are frustrated or angry.

- *Piss-takers.* Meaning people who abuse you or take your energy.

- *Taking the piss.* Denotes making fun of something/someone or when someone is abusing or taking advantage of a situation.

- *Pissing on my bonfire/fireworks.* Means your fun and joy are taken away.

- *Pissing on your grave.* Denotes being totally disrespected.

- *Getting or being pissed.* Being totally drunk, so out-of-control, vulnerable.

- *Wee! Yippee!* The sound we make when we slide or are playful, a 'happy' wee.

- *Having a slash.* Means urinating, being slashed, cuts like a knife.

- *I'm piss-poor.* Denotes poverty, when Victorians sold their urine.

- *I don't have a pot to piss in.* Being vulnerable poor, negative energy to wee.

- *Piss off.* Telling someone to go away as they irritate you.

- *Being on the piss.* Means either getting drunk or being wonky/imbalanced.

- *Being in a pissy mood.* Denotes being angry or irritable.

- *Peeved.* Indicates being irritated or annoyed.

- *Pissed/peed my pants.* Means you got really scared/were terrified.

- *I'll have a P, please, Bob.* The UK saying making a joke about needing to pee.

- *I can feel it in my waters/waterworks.* Intuition, knowing something deeply.

- *Oh, here come the waterworks.* Meaning manipulating with emotions/crying.

- *I wouldn't piss on you if you were on fire.* Signs of deeply hating someone.

- *Go with the flow/against the flow.* Means allowing a situation or resisting it.

- *Being or getting bladdered.* Denotes being drunk, filling up with alcohol.

- *Piss-ant.* An insult used in the USA.

- *Pissing in the wind.* Doing something that is a waste of time or ineffective.

*Can you think of any more in your culture or language?*

We used to be more aware of energy and the world around us and within us, we were more metaphysical. For those unfamiliar with metaphysics, which just means 'beyond physics' or beyond the physical realm, everything is energy vibrating at different frequencies, resulting in a variety of shapes, sizes or density.

Similar frequencies hang around together engaging in the law of attraction, what I call '**energy begets similar energy**'.

**Emotions also relate to similar energies to our body parts.**

Given the clues in the language, the frequencies of frustration, holding stuff in, or abuse, especially sexual or bullying, is similar to the energy of our bladder. Therefore, if we do not deal with the emotional or mental issues that piss us off, or if we allow people to take the piss, it will eventually affect the bladder because that is where those undealt emotions reside.

*Taking the piss* means when someone negatively messing with someone else or taking advantage of them.

**There is only so much crap that we can sweep under the carpet before it starts to bulge and trip us up.**

If you are someone who uses humour to hide behind instead of dealing with the root cause of an issue, you may also be damaging your bladder, as well as other organs.

If you laugh when someone disrespects you in a way to diffuse it, hide behind, make them stop, and worst still, if you end up accepting their behaviour, allowing that frequency of piss-taker in, and then taking the piss out of yourself, you are storing this energy in your bladder. The long-term effect may result in physical urinary issues.

These will not be identified by the medical world and most therapists won't find anything wrong with you either, but it doesn't mean there isn't. It just means that modern science, no matter how amazing and at times life-saving, has not yet caught up with nature, and inventors have not yet fathomed a way to prove certain things, but that doesn't mean they do not exist.

Taking back control of communicating honestly with your body and being more aware of basic metaphysics and how you can use it to benefit your health is a huge step in your wellbeing, and to having a happy bladder.

I did warn you in the beginning that this was an extensive look at all options to help bladders, right?

Awesome. Let's continue then.

**The following illustration shows us how our physical body is linked to our mental, emotional and spiritual body, and how we also have chakras and meridians. We are more than a physical being.**

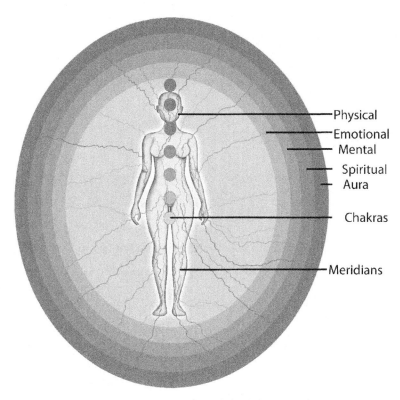

Physical
Emotional
Mental
Spiritual
Aura

Chakras

Meridians

Copyright Dr Jennifer Meyer

**Metaphysical treatment example:**

During a personal development weekend, I performed a crystal reiki healing session on a client. This entailed her lying down in silence, resting with me being present and connecting mentally with her psyche and aura, putting my hands over her body to feel the energy of her chakras. I placed relevant crystals on and around her body and used them to increase the healing frequency from my hands. I mention it here as it is a clear example of metaphysics at work in health matters.

She referred to the treatment as *life-changing*.

Her body's energy indicated to me to help her stomach at the metaphysical level, so emotions dealing with bullying, loss of personal power, feeling sick, nervous. I tuned into her aura and saw her at a desk at work, shrivelled up. Then I saw straws from her solar plexus connecting to co-workers. So, workplace bullying and hating her job were sucking her power and allowing bullies to drain her further.

Then I saw the colours blue and purple, indicating the ears area, at which point Archangel Michael appeared and said he had been talking to her, but she was not listening. The ringing in her ears is him telling her she is destined to change jobs and work with the angels by becoming a therapist and helping people and the answer is *yes* – she keeps asking if it's the right time. He and his angels will be there if she takes the first step. He left a gift in her aura, I had no idea what as it was none of my business, just to relay the message to the client.

I cleared what stuck energy I could and provided healing, as did the crystals, and then I passed on the information. She said she wasn't expecting messages, just a treatment but the information was life-changing. She burst into tears explaining how she hated her bullying boss, colleagues and her job to the point where she makes herself sick.

She was gobsmacked that I mentioned Archangel Michael as she had been praying to him and hadn't told anyone that she was thinking of training in angel therapy.

She skipped out of the session, somehow I reckon she quit her job not long after that.

Do not underestimate the level of healing and information that metaphysicians can help you with.

**Note:** as in any industry, there are charlatans masking as metaphysicians, there are therapists that are not qualified or that don't have much experience. There are some that are true and natural. Things to ask or look out for, where they trained, how much experience they have practising, which governing body or associations they belong to in their trade, and do they have insurance. Sometimes a natural won't need any official training, they are born gifted and crafted that skill, and that's OK too.

The more present you are, the more you listen to your senses, the more you will know which therapist is right for you and which treatments will best help you.

### Visualisation Aid

A bladder can be seen as a bagpipe. The main ball is the bladder, which deflates when empty and expands when full. The skin contracts in and out when in play. It has tubes, one for the mouth and others coming out of the bag. Your bladder is the bag and the air is the urine and the mouth tube is your mouth. The start of your digestive tract and the other tubes are the exit where the air comes out, so in the bladder's case, the urethra. If the pipes are not properly attached, air leaks. If the stitching around the bag is loose, air leaks. If there is a blockage in the pipes or the bag, it won't work. The same with our bladder, we need to look after it.

Our bladder, like all organs, is crucial to our health. It has a unique sound and plays a role in the orchestra that is our whole being.

This book is mainly about that instrument, but if a note is perfect, it will then have a ripple effect on all the orchestra and therefore a happy bladder means a happier body, and an even happier you.

**Energy begets similar energy.** If you are often angry you will attract things to make you angrier. If you feel and believe you are lucky or blessed, you will attract wonders.

Waterworks, bladders, water, and urine are all linked to the element of water and the water elementals called Undines, water spirits or nymphs.

More on this in the metaphysical protocol: I'm just sowing another seed.

## Chapter 3 Keynotes

- The bladder forms part of our urinary tract and digestive system.

- The bladder is a holding station, a bag to keep urine until it can be released.

- The ureters are one-way tubes passing urine from the kidneys to the bladder.

- The urethra is the tube linking the bladder to your precious holes area, where urine exits the body.

- A woman has 3 precious holes: urethra, vagina, and anus.

- A man has 2 precious holes: urethra and anus.

- I class the pelvic area as the bladder, womb, ovaries, fallopian tubes, vagina, lower intestines, colon, pelvis, hips. (prostate, scrotum, penis).

- Energy begets similar energy. The power of attraction. Like attracts like.

- Metaphysics plays a vital role in bladder health.

- Clues are in our language. Any phrase using the words: bladder, piss, pee, wee, pipi, pee-pee, slash, urine, flow, whizz, or waterworks has an energy link to our bladder.

## Action! Interactive bit, it's your turn:

1. What two things strike you the most from this chapter?

2. Can you think of when you were really taken the piss out of (when someone disrespected you, took advantage or teased you)?

When you got pissed off, and didn't do anything to clear those energies out? And, can you link it to having a bout of any type of cystitis? It doesn't matter if you can't, we are slowly opening up doors that have been sealed shut.

3. Draw your own precious holes in your journal to help understand your female anatomy. Ensure you have properly looked at yourself in the mirror, in case you omitted to do that before. I realise for some of you that is hard to do and you may feel weird or even perverse, I did at first, but it is totally natural.

So, we have learnt about **our waterworks**.

We understand that we have **precious holes** and **flaps** surrounding them.

We are now familiar with basic metaphysics and how feelings and trapped issues at the mental, emotional, and spiritual levels will affect the physical, and we know that there are clues in our language about the bladder linking emotions or lifestyle.

Let's not dilly-dally and get moving onto another crucial section: why does cystitis happen?

Remember those cystitis types we mentioned in chapter two?

Well, it's time to go deep diving into those.

Deep breath.

Go.

# CHAPTER 4

# Why Cystitis Happens

Let's go through the different types of cystitis in-depth and how they come about.

Remember, the gold is in the details. It is a good idea to build on what we learn, therefore, repetition is useful.

You have already seen these types laid out like this in chapter two, so it will help the deeper information sink in better.

*Bear with me again, this is a long chapter and we get technical, so feel free to go get a cuppa now and cruise on through. We've got this.*

Start realising how to avoid getting each type, as we understand how they could come about, just do the opposite, in other words, avoid doing the things that could trigger that type of cystitis. We will then add to that by exploring the *protocols* in part two.

## Type 1: Interstitial Cystitis (IC/BPS)

This condition is most likely caused by:

- A flaw in bladder tissue allowing irritating elements in pee to penetrate the walls.

- An inflammatory cell (mast cell) producing histamine and other substances that lead to cystitis symptoms similar to autoimmune diseases.

- Sugary, infected, or over-concentrated pee upsetting the bladder walls.

- Problems in the nerves responsible for bladder senses causing pain as a result of normal functions such as the bladder filling with pee and storing it.

- An overactive immune system attacking the bladder, like other autoimmune conditions.

- The tenderness in the pelvic area can worsen with core muscle exercises.

- Any type of stress, especially chronic stress, will contribute to this condition.

- Inflammatory foods too much acidity: sugar, tomatoes, coffee, chocolate, gluten, dairy, alcohol, spicy, peppers, sweeteners, chemicals/pesticides.

- Blocked energies related to bladder frequencies, see 'metaphysical cystitis'.

Sometimes it can suddenly come on (like an allergy) and stay for a few months and then disappear. In some cases, it stays for years or longer.

**Bladder ulcers** also called 'Hunner's lesions/patches' are part of IC (interstitial cystitis) and are not the same ulcers that you get elsewhere. They are specific patches of inflammation on the bladder wall related to IC.

## Type 2: Bacterial Infection/UTI

There are two ways of getting an infection in the bladder.

### 1: Internally

A germ through your digestive track ending up irritating the bladder walls. The body reacts by protecting itself, creating inflammation and producing more cystitis symptoms. Two common nasty bacteria that can cause cystitis are Streptococcus and E.Coli.

Sometimes the germ may settle first in the kidneys, creating a kidney infection (a urinary tract infection could mean kidneys, ureters, bladder, or urethra) and will usually travel down to the bladder too. It is possible to have a bladder infection without affecting the kidneys.

### 2: Externally

You can also catch a bacterial infection, and this is the most common way, from the outside. When bacteria travel up the urethra and settle onto the bladder walls. So a germ can get into the bladder via the ureters from the kidneys (internally) or via the urethra (externally) from your vulva area. There are several ways bacteria can touch your urethra, for example, through sex, masturbation, dirty sex toys, bad toilet hygiene, tight underwear, tampons left in too long, or splashback from the dirty water in the toilet bowl, just to name a few. Much more on that later.

## Type 3: Candida Cystitis

Candida is also known as thrush, fungus, yeast, or the 'bad gut bacteria'. Usually, Candida lives in our intestines, where it should, providing it is in balance with our 'good gut bacteria'. It forms part of our microbiome (our internal floral ecosystem), but if we have too much food and drink that feed the yeast, it will over-flourish and spread, killing off the good flora and migrating outside of the gut walls, a 'leaky gut'.

There are two ways into the bladder, internally via the ureters, or externally via the urethra.

**Internally**

So, yes we can absolutely get candida in our bladder by eating certain foods or from a leaky gut. If we have candida issues in our gut or mouth, the likelihood is we also have it in the bladder.

A bladder is moist, dark, and cramped when empty, providing a thriving environment for candida. Getting rid of it takes some effort, but it is necessary.

When I approached my urologist with this idea, he poo-pooed it mumbling,

'No such thing as candida'.

It was a taboo, something not accepted in medical terms. Now it is more mainstream, although I still have not heard a medic suggest we have candida in the bladder.

If you take away one thing from this book, it is that this type of cystitis does exist.

**You can have candida or thrush inside your bladder.**

This type does not show up in a urine or blood test. The only way to know for sure is with a camera procedure. As I have been through this, you can identify it by yourself too, by analysing your diet and doing the detox that worked for me.

The good news is that once the candida has died, the symptoms will go away and it will have to grow again to be problematic. I will teach you later how to listen to your body's signals so you can counteract new candida spores from flourishing.

**Externally**

The other way to get thrush in your bladder is from the outside. If you have thrush in your vagina, or anus, a burning sensation that makes your bits swell up and itch, there is a high risk that some of that thrush will transfer into the urethra.

This is common, especially in women with precious holes that are closer together.

The risk increases by wearing strings/thongs or tight trousers.

You don't have to have vaginal thrush to get it in your bladder as it can also be transferred sexually, if your partner has it or has been touching someone that does before sleeping with you, or if you have been with someone and then touch yourself. You can avoid 'contact candida' by implementing the sexual protocols, toilet protocols, and daily hygiene protocols, coming up later.

Beware of introducing food or drink on your lady-bits or your partner's penis. I know a girl whose partner wanted to use strawberry yoghurt during oral sex, this could also be chocolate spread or anything else that has no business touching your vulva, and that will be licked and pushed up all your precious holes. She got vaginal thrush and cystitis within 48 hours. The sugar and chemicals in these products will encourage candida and irritate the skin so your holes will swell up to stop the intrusion, and if any is in the urethra already, then the swelling may push it up into the bladder. I will go into detail in the 'sexual cystitis' type.

## Type 4: Viral Infection

Please see type 2, as catching a viral infection is pretty much the same as catching a bacterial one. A viral infection is caused by a virus, like catching a cold, or getting the flu, but this virus prefers to settle in the kidneys or the bladder.

The stronger your immune system, the less chance a virus will affect you.

If you get ill a lot you may wish to be tested via a blood test for a 'silent' virus that can live in you for decades. It is called Epstein-Barr Virus, EBV. This virus is common if you have had glandular fever or chronic fatigue. I call it silent as sometimes it is partly responsible for many ailments that we blame other stuff for. It can be linked with thyroid issues, urinary issues, fatigue, auto-immune diseases and much more. It is worth asking for a blood test to check for past and present infections. There are some antiviral treatments possible if you have it. Great nutrition avoiding things that feed it is also a good idea. It feeds on similar foods to candida, so basically what I class as non-foods, but it also loves eggs, so in addition to cutting out other problematic foods I would cut out eggs too whilst you have EBV.

I have had EBV and it did affect my bladder.

## Type 5: Metaphysical Cystitis

We are not just our physical body. We have thoughts, belief patterns, ideas, moral codes, dreams, aspirations, a vast array of emotions, spiritual understanding and connections, faith, secrets, and traumas, at all levels. We are more than a physical body, which is the realm that is dealt with by the medical world.

**We are a mosaic of different energies.**

Energy vibrates at different frequencies. In a simple way, *everything* is energy. So everything (inanimate or alive) has a frequency that denotes its shape, colour, solidity, and function.

Even though at the smallest level, everything is made from the same source energy, uniqueness is defined by frequency resonance.

We are all the same and yet unique. The way our energies form our body, including mind, spirit, emotions, aura, is unique, as is our DNA, and yet also interconnected.

We will attract energy resonating at any level of similar frequency to us.

This is called *the law of attraction.*

Each of our body-parts has its own frequency, remember the orchestra analogy, all form the same band, all needed to produce a beautiful harmonious song, but all very different. A bassoonist is different from a pianist. A bladder is not like a tooth. Agreed?

OK, so our bladder vibrates at a certain energy level and can, therefore, act as a beacon for similar frequencies that are compatible energy-wise, but not health-wise.

What may surprise you, is what frequencies are similar to bladders, some of these will also vibrate with other organs, such as anger with the liver, loss and grief with the lungs and heart, but all the following vibrate to bladder frequencies.

- Frustration

- Irritation

- Pissed-off-ness

- Piss-takers, Piss-taking

- Holding on to things emotionally/or physically by hoarding

- Fear, terror

- Being too nice/People-Pleaser

- Secrets related to certain abuse, especially sexual or toxic substances

- Disconnection from safety or what we consider to be our home

- Despair

- Self-loathing

- Living someone else's life

- Inauthenticity

- Sarcasm used to destroy the self

- Fake laughter

- A belief pattern of poverty or desolation

- Trapped in a social bubble that you don't resonate with

- Cave-diving trauma and to some extent scuba diving issues

- Certain emotional traumas related to the element of water, our psyche, and emotional bodies, which is another reason why we call our urinary tract system our *Waterworks.*

- Going against the flow

- Poverty complex or belief you are and always will be too poor

- Secondary, where emotional and mental blocks started elsewhere and festered and have since been transferred physically to the bladder.

So, if you have experienced any of these energies from childhood, or are still hanging on to traumas, or if you were sexually assaulted and have not dealt with these issues effectively, then eventually these may affect your bladder, because they have similar frequencies and can interconnect, like fitting a male plug into a female ended one: it just clicks.

Any unresolved issues at any unseen body's levels – emotional, mental, or spiritual– can have ripple effects and affect our physical body too. Vice versa, if you have a physical trauma that is not dealt with or that lasts a long time, or even permanently, this will affect the related frequencies in the metaphysical realm.

All metaphysical means, remember, is 'beyond physical'.

'Metaphysical cystitis' is not identified or recognised by the medical world, and that is where there is a huge gap in understanding how our bodies work and how things can affect our bladders. We are going to spend quite a while in this section, as this is just as crucial as the physical.

We are complex beings so we need to explore our deeper levels to fully understand our bladder.

Take a moment to think about if any of the related unresolved issues, previously mentioned, have affected you at some point in your life.

**Are you a chronic 'people-pleaser'? If so, you may wish to reconsider.**

People who are 'too nice' can get cystitis metaphysically because they let themselves get taken the piss out of and don't speak their truth, it can also affect their throat and mouth, but that is a discussion for another book.

Anything that you sweep under the carpet will create a monster. If some of those things relate to the bladder frequency, they will end up energetically in the bladder.

**This won't show up in a scan as it is energy not matter, but trust me, it does matter.**

All **energetic toxins** will affect you as much as physical toxins. To be free from dis-ease, we need to understand everything that can throw us off balance: metaphysical influence is huge.

The physical part of our body is the tip of the iceberg. If you leave your health, be it physical or mental, only to the doctors, you may never be free of disease and remain at their mercy.

The purpose of this book is to illuminate *all* that affects the bladder so you can look after yourself better at *all* levels. This may include employing help from good doctors, specialists, surgeons, holistic therapists, counsellors, priests, life coaches, and more helpers *if* needed, but this book is putting you back in the driver's seat.

*Allow this information to sink in, re-read it now with an even more open mind.*

Trust that your body knows everything, it is the wisest being on the planet and this information is resonating in your sub-consciousness, awakening a deeper connection with your bladder.

Energy can be altered by just an awareness of it.

Observing energy changes it. So, just by reading about metaphysical issues to do with your bladder, you have already started a healing process.

Start increasing that healing by having relevant holistic treatments during your bladder health journey. I will go into that in the 'metaphysical protocols' section.

## Type 6: Overactive Bladder (OAB)/ Urgency Urinary Incontinence (UUI)

An overactive bladder is when your bladder can no longer hold in the pee. You suddenly need to wee without any warning. This could lead to peeing yourself involuntarily, which is a type of incontinence. It is an overly *keen* bladder, *ooh look a drop of pee, let's evacuate it right now!* And you could also be just producing a lot of urine, needing to pee way more often than usual.

There are many reasons or potential causes of OAB such as:
a weak, impaired or spasming bladder-wall muscle ( the detrusor muscle); neurologic condition; diabetes; being overweight; pregnancy; childbirth; menopause; hormone issues; drinking far too much liquid in one day; taking medication for urine production; UTI; consuming bladder irritating food or drinks; not emptying your bladder fully; bladder stones or abnormalities.

## Type 7: Stress Urinary Incontinence (SUI)

Stress urinary incontinence is due to a weakened urethra where it can no longer take the weight/pressure of the urine in the bladder, and the sphincter doesn't quite close properly. It results in peeing yourself through physical stress. This could be as a result of sneezing, coughing, laughing, lifting heavy objects, bending, exercising or walking. This is also is due to weakened pelvic floor muscles. There are many ways to weaken these muscles, such as a sedentary lifestyle, smoking, being overweight, and coughing for too long due to illness, pregnancy, childbirth, nerve injuries, or surgery in the pelvic area.

## Type 8: Overflow Incontinence

If the bladder has a blockage or stones, or the sphincter or urethra is blocked in any way, then pee will escape and go around the obstacle, resulting in peeing yourself involuntarily. This could also happen if for some reason (usually nerve signalling issue) your brain does not register that you need to pee, then the bladder gets over-full and the urine has to push its way out as it has nowhere else to go. Think of it as a balloon that you fill with water, at some point, it will either burst or leak out of the knot you are holding. Blockages or stones happen for many reasons, mainly dehydration, too many toxins in the concentrated urine, not evacuating your pee fully, or you could have cancer or cysts in your bladder or urethra.

## Type 9: Functional Incontinence

There are so many reasons why we do not go to the toilet when we need to. It could be because we are disabled and cannot get to a toilet on time, it could be due to pain such as arthritis not allowing us enough time to get to the loo. It could be dementia not remembering where the loo is or being confused. It could be due to depression and "letting yourself go". It could be as a result of anxiety, stress or bullying or that you just can't go in public toilets or have people know or see you go to the loo. You could also be frightened and pee yourself through fear. It could be you are too scared of the dark to get up at night, or you need to go to the loo but are dreaming that you are peeing and so actually wet the bed.

{Why Cystitis Happens | 99}

We can also class **Bedwetting** in this class of incontinence.

If you experience more than one type, this is classed as **Mixed Incontinence.**

Having all types of urinary incontinence, or one type but where you have zero control over your urine, this is called **Total Incontinence.**

## Type 10: Irritable Bladder Syndrome (IBS)

If you suffer from IBS in the intestines, you are likely to have it in the bladder too at some point. You can get IBS (bladder) without IBS (bowels).

You can also get this due to certain foods and drinks that irritate your bladder. Remember, that what you eat, drink, inhale, or touch may end up caressing your bladder walls, so please be mindful.

Some people are more sensitive to certain foods than others. Some are coeliac (allergic to gluten), some have diabetes and are more affected by sugars, and some cannot tolerate beyond a certain amount of irritable foods and drinks.

These could be the same foods that react with your bowels. These foods can vary depending on the person. This is where you need to keep a record of everything you eat and drink and be precise with it.

Write everything that passes your lips for at least two weeks, and also track your symptoms.

See if you can notice a pattern. For example, when I have cranberry juice or those cystitis sachets, I have cramps or a burning sensation when I pee within 4 hours. I know some cystitis sufferers cannot tolerate olive oil, although I'm absolutely fine with it, and they seem OK with cranberry juice.

Even in IC or IBS sufferers, there will be differences. I'm now OK with gluten and certain sugars but at one point I could not even have the tiniest amount. Some people can have alcohol with IC, and some not.

**It is important to listen to *your* body and not someone else's.**

Make a list of your trigger foods and drinks. Remember sensitivity is personal, so if someone you know can eat and drink the same food and they don't suffer, it doesn't make it OK for you.

IBS is your body communicating to you the best way it knows, to stop eating a specific food or drink that it deems as toxic.

Imagine giving a toddler a Brussel-sprout, you know the videos on the internet when they screw up their face, throw a hissy fit, launching the offensive food on the floor, red-faced, and angered. It is obvious that the baby is not enjoying that food and does not want it. Our bladder tells us the same thing, but we don't always listen.

If you think you have a sensitive bladder, or IBS either bladder or bowels, then eliminate some or all these potential triggers and see how you feel.

This list is also what to remove if you have candida, as these foods are inflammatory, meaning they cause inflammation, make your body over-acidic and feed the candida.

**Common trigger foods and drinks:**

- Sugar, any type including fruit, honey and cranberry

- Sweeteners, any type especially aspartame

- Additives, chemicals, E-numbers

- Dairy, all types

- Gluten

- Corn

- Eggs

- Peanuts

- Cashews

- Nightshades: potatoes, peppers, aubergine, tomatoes

- Cauliflower

- Some spices, especially chilli

- Ice-cold food or drink

- Alcohol

- Fizzy drinks

- Yeast, fungus or fermented foods such as blue cheese, mushrooms, soy sauce, yoghurt-health drinks.

- Caffeine

- Chocolate

- Tobacco/Nicotine

I understand that this list is daunting and giving up all these foods that you love. It doesn't have to be forever, but just whilst you are identifying your trigger foods.

Once your bladder has detoxed from them, you can slowly re-introduce one at a time, to see if the intolerance has gone. I will elaborate in the 'nutrition protocols'.

**Note:** for IBS as in Irritable BOWEL Syndrome, raw veggies, onion, and garlic can also be a trigger, although not necessarily for IBS Irritable Bladder Syndrome.

## Type 11: Sexual Cystitis

This includes sex with a partner, either male or female, several partners, or sex with yourself so masturbation.

We will cover this section in-depth as I know of many women who don't enjoy sex, due to fear of getting ill with either thrush or cystitis. So get comfortable, we are going in!

Sexual cystitis can be just that, an inflamed bladder and general pelvic area swelling as a result of sex, even if the sexual hygiene protocols were properly followed.

So, a common reason why women get cystitis is through sex.

SEX is a huge trigger for sexual, bacterial, viral or candida cystitis.

This is because the penis, tongue, fingers, toys, vegetables (no judgement here!), are direct delivery systems for germs, thrush, bacteria, and foreign bodies, into where it has no business being, so your mouth, your womb, your colon, and unfortunately, your poor bladder.

Mechanically speaking, sex involves a lot of trauma. I'm not talking about any mental anguish, guilt, emotional trauma or abuse, although I will touch upon those in the metaphysical section.

I'm talking here about the physical impact of two bodies pumping each other.

Look at your hands. They feel OK, comfortable. Now, rub them together vigorously, you will feel friction and burning. Clap them together as hard as you can for a minute (or the length of time you have sex!) and now what? They hurt. They may even feel swollen and battered because they are.

Now, imagine the delicate skin of your precious holes being bashed continuously by your partner's pelvic area and wiry pubes, if he has them. I agree it may feel good at the time, thanks to sex hormones and endorphins, but it is still a traumatic event for that area.

The weight of the partner thrusting upon you also impacts your internal pelvic area. Sex, no matter how gentle, is going to end up in some sort of inflammation, it is a natural reaction the body has when being under attack or pressure.

Imagine shutting your fingers in a car door. Ouch. What happens? They swell up, for many reasons, but one reason is for self-protection, cushioning the affected area, like wrapping it up in bubble-wrap or a comforting hug after a boo-boo.

Your body will do the same thing with your inner and outer pelvic area after sex.

So, as I said, even if it does not develop into another type of cystitis, it is possible to suffer symptoms of cystitis or urethritis after sex. Remember, cystitis just means a swollen bladder. Sex may irritate, causing inflammation in your pelvic area, including the precious holes, bladder, colon, and womb. In most people, it doesn't bother them, but with those who are prone to cystitis or vaginal dryness, it may.

I'm not saying don't have sex. I'm explaining it mechanically so it will be easier to understand when I describe the sexual protocols for 'bladder-safe sex'.

Sexual cystitis is why after sex it can be hard to pee, it trickles out shyly because your urethra is swollen and pee is struggling to get passed. It may only last for a while and not develop into anything more, but nevertheless it is a type of cystitis, or at least pelvic-itis, meaning swelling of any parts of your lady-bits on the inside (tubes, womb, bladder, colon, hips) and on the outside (vagina, urethra, rectum, thighs and skin).

A dirty partner or a dirty anything used for sexual pleasure is problematic.

**Pubic Hair**

Think of Mr Twit's beard (The Roald Dahl character), and what lives in it.

Imagine that beard as your partner's pubic area, rubbing against the delicate skin of your precious holes: ew.

Same for men with facial hair during oral sex. You know how sore your lips and chin can be after a good snogging-session with a bearded or bristly man, now think of your vulva skin, it is delicate and soft and may be insulted by facial or pubic hair.

Your own pubic hair or your partner's can be a nest for bacteria, thrush, or lice and due to proximity to the urethra can transfer things up there.

Even if clean, pubes and beards can be problematic. Some beards are soft and cause much less irritation, but that stubble or prickly beard can be a trigger if they rummage around your precious holes too long.

Some people said to me when I studied this, that it is natural to have pubic hair.

Yes, it is, but our bodies take millions of years to adapt to our environmental changes, so when humans first existed, any body hair was crucial to keep warm as we had not yet invented clothes or central heating.

Survival meant water, food, warmth, and sex, to procreate, a natural urge built in us. So it was important to keep the testes and scrotum warm in a man to encourage good healthy semen. It was important for women to have a warm vulva so that the vaginal cavity didn't sew itself back up in the cold (slight exaggeration, but I like the imagery) and would be welcoming to the penis.

Protection is why we have hair on our armpits, to nurture our lymph system. There are major points in our lymph glands in our groin (another reason for pubes there) and in our armpits (hence hair there) keeping them warm, and also to trap any toxins coming out in sweat or urine.

We have moved on since then as we have showers, hygiene knowledge, clothing, and deodorant, although don't get me started on aluminium salts and aerosols, I will keep that for the 'products' chapter.

So, yes, our ancestors did need body hair, but we don't. So it is up to you, but if you are a cystitis sufferer, then I recommend waxing your pubic area, or shaving if you are not quite brave enough for the 'Hollywood', a full vaginal area wax, ouch, but so worth it.

And yes, I do.

## Oral Sex

Poor oral hygiene, either in you or your partner, may also affect your vulva health.

For example, you go out for a meal and some alcohol (sugar, acid, germs) and then kiss someone (their sugar, acid, germs, alcohol, tobacco and anyone they kissed before you). You have oral sex before the main entertainment, and boom. Anything living in your mouth or your partner's mouth is now potentially travelling up the urethra to the bladder. Sometimes we get away with it, sometimes we don't, either way, each time you have *any* type of sex, your bladder is at risk.

## Anal Sex

This is a common reason to get bacterial and candida cystitis. Remember that some candida is present, quite rightly, in the gut and hence the colon. The colon is where we poo from, so think about what lives there and on the rectum walls: faecal matter, even if microscopic; gut bacteria from the floral ecosystem; candida; toxins, what the body has already deemed as no good for us; bad bacteria or possible infection.

So, if you do enjoy anal sex, be aware that there are ways to counteract this in the sexual protocols in the next chapter. So, anything going in or out of your butt will affect your vulva area, remember that our 3 precious holes are close together.

Let's imagine (no, this isn't a porno, I promise!) that in the throes of passion, your partner slips his finger in your bum, then pulls it out and puts in your vagina, and then continues caressing the vulva area.

You get the picture, classic transference. No getting away from it, minuscule bits of poo, bacteria, fungus, and toxins are now inside your vagina and smeared over your urethra, as well as anything else lurking under his fingernails.

Now, add the thrusting factor, so his hand or penis pumping your precious area for quite some time (if you are lucky), ensuring that the germ, or whatever microscopic thing that has no business being there, is now pushed directly into your womb and up your urethra.

Result? Hello, good sex, goodbye bladder and vaginal health. Hello, days of soreness and unfortunately, a type of cystitis and/or vaginal thrush.

If this happens most times that you have sex, then the metaphysical aspect comes into play, and you develop a belief system or a mental pattern that dictates that with each new partner, or anytime that you have sex, you will get ill, and so you almost set that up before sex begins, making it more likely to happen, as the law of attraction takes hold, more on the metaphysics later.

This transference method does also concern men. Not as much for the one receiving anal, as their urethra opening is far from their anus, but that said, for the giver, it is problematic. Imagine male anal sex or male inside a woman's butt, his urethra is touching his partner's colon walls where all *that* stuff lives and with the thrusting, having a good rummage, pushing stuff up his own urethra. The reason men are less likely to get bacterial, candida or viral cystitis is because they have a longer urethra than women, and so are more likely to pee the germs out before they reach the bladder, but it is still very much a factor to look out for.

There is a further chance of transference for both partners after penetration, as licking and kissing occur. Remember, what you put in your mouth may affect your bladder eventually. So, an infection of sorts could then be introduced internally.

## Menstruation/Period

This isn't about sex but a great place to mention other triggers of transference which are tampons and sanitary towels.

So, remember, anything that touches or enters your pelvic region can impact your urethra and hence the bladder.

### I once got a UTI due to a tampon.

I have had bacterial cystitis when I left my tampon in too long. Remember anything but fresh wee has no business touching bladder walls. I know you do not stick a tampon up your urethra! Thank goodness! Yet the string on a tampon does touch the urethra, and so do your hands and any germs on them, whilst applying or removing the tampon. Any sweat, blood, or pee leaches onto a tampon or tampon-string and lingers around your precious holes.

You get the idea. The same thing with a sanitary towel, the material of it may irritate your vulva area, so try using organic cotton pads, or use a clean 'Moon-Cup' (a rubber cup inserted into the vagina to collect blood and them emptied) more on that in hygiene protocols and products section.

So, if you do use tampons or towels then change them frequently with clean hands.

### I sincerely vote against tampons of any kind, ever.

Having sex during a period could bring on cystitis. The area is already swollen due to menstruation, so adding sexual activity and possible transfer of old blood to the urethra is not a great idea for those prone to cystitis.

Sexual health and hygiene are crucial in general not just for bladder health, and I'm assuming you are aware of that, for in this book I am concentrating on the bladder, after all, I promised you that in the title, but do remember that our body parts are all connected and so the more you can do to keep all your body healthy and hygienic, the happier your bladder will be. If we remember that the bladder is a dude in a great orchestra, he wants the rest of the team on their A-game, creating harmonious music.

**Note:** cystitis is not a sexually transmitted disease, but dirty sex can be the cause of sexual, candida, viral and bacterial infection cystitis.

## Type 12: Medically Induced Cystitis/Iatrogenic

This inflammation or irritation is a direct result of medical intervention, such as surgery. Obviously cutting and disturbing this area will irritate the bladder or other places in the area the operation takes place.

The dye for an MRI going in via an injection into your bloodstream is used to illuminate fluid going through our urinary tract. This causes upset whilst it travels through and you will feel a weird sensation, like heat and burning and instant cystitis. This tends to go away not long after the procedure once you have a wee.

A camera in the urethra and up the bladder will irritate as it touches the lining on the way up and down and also the walls and more so if biopsies are taken.

The numbing gel inserted into the urethra and bladder for a cystoscopy.

This numbing chemical in the gel produces an instant feeling of burning and that irritable symptom of cystitis. It does go away after drinking plenty of water to flush it out, but it can last up to 24 hours.

The use of catheters will most likely also cause offence as the tubes and sphincter are forced open, causing urethritis and possible cystitis, although medically necessary, there are ways to avoid catheter-induced cystitis, as mentioned earlier.

## Type 13: Pregnancy

Cystitis can be common during pregnancy. As the baby grows, it expands the womb taking up more than its usual share of the pelvic area, affecting its neighbouring organs, the bladder or the bowels. The womb pushes against the bladder creating a pressure that will irritate it. It may make you feel weird and make you want to pee more often. Pregnancy and childbirth can be causes of urinary incontinence.

Our body goes through a lot of chemical and hormonal fluctuations during pregnancy and so that is another factor that may cause cystitis and other issues such as vomiting, morning sickness, weight gain, tiredness and the list goes on.

For a natural process, pregnancy can come with a plethora of problems.

## Type 14: Abnormal Pressure Cystitis

Any lump in the pelvic region may also aggravate the bladder. So anything pushing the bladder or growing in the pelvic area (womb, ovaries, urinary tract, colon, intestines, testes or prostate), such as cysts, fibroids, ulcers, stones, lumps or cancer may produce cystitis symptoms, including pressure, an irritating sensation, or the frequent need to pee.

## Type 15: Leucoplakia Cystitis

As we know this is a mucosal disease showing up as white patches and lesions on the bladder walls. Medical science has not really done too much research on this, and leucoplakia in the urinary tract is considered rare, however, I had it, so don't let rarity put you off getting checked for this if you have the symptoms.

You need a camera in the bladder and possible biopsies of the tissue to identify it. Medically there doesn't seem to be any treatments, I certainly wasn't offered any, although this can be a premalignant condition, so it is advised to have it diagnosed and followed up regularly. The symptoms are typical cystitis, so painful pee, uncomfortable pelvic area, urge to pee frequently, difficulty peeing, blood in urine, abdominal bloating, and sometimes white bits in the urine and frequent UTI's.

I cannot identify why I got this but I found that ridding myself of candida and following a strict diet of no sugars or alcohol helped. Smoking is linked to leucoplakia in the mouth, so definitely give up smoking if you have any leucoplakia in your body.

The urologist who found the leucoplakia in my bladder (Dr Beep-Head) was arrogant and did not tell me anything about the condition other than it is not really researched and not to worry about it.

Don't be fooled! It is a condition that may promote cancer and it is not supposed to be in your bladder, so insist on having biopsies and be followed every six months until it has gone, or if it gets worse and if cancer cells start appearing then it can be dealt with sooner if you know about it.

At the time I didn't realise leucoplakia denoted possible pre-cancerous conditions so I didn't insist on being followed or treated and was dismissed by the medical world, which encouraged me to do my own research, eventually resulting in this book.

Stand up, be loud and *insist* to be checked regularly if you have this condition. Don't let arrogant or misinformed medics dismiss you. If your urologist is difficult, sack him and get a second opinion.

Leucoplakia *is* a big deal.

## Type 16: Menopausal Cystitis

Once we start the menopause we release less and less oestrogen (our female hormones linked to reproduction, lubrication and so many other things).

If you go through the menopause at a natural age about 50+ it may not cause too many concerns. If you have it early say before 45 or premature so before 40, it probably will.

Amongst many other factors of menopausal symptom, it can cause cystitis and urethritis. This is due to dryness as a lack of natural lubrication and hormone fluctuations. Most women suffer from vaginal dryness, however, in cystitis sufferers, this may also be urethra dryness. The skin inside will be dry and causes symptoms of burning after pee and general discomfort in that area.

One way to help this is to go on HRT (with your doctor's approval and being followed regularly, being fully aware of all the side-effects and risks). If you do not wish to go on HRT then you can get prescribed oestrogen in a pessary that you insert inside your vagina and this will help to lubricate your precious holes from within.

A pessary is a localised application of hormones and therefore may have fewer potential risks or side-effects than HRT taken orally or from patches. The oestrogen in the pessary will seep into the vaginal walls and therefore lubricate the urethra too. As with any medication, it is crucial to talk to your doctor about the benefits and risks and make the decision if going on medication is right for you at that time.

Never insert anything into your urethra, unless you have a medical procedure and in the hands of a good doctor or urologist.

You can also lubricate the outside of your precious holes area (your flaps) with an approved lubricant or moisturiser but again never put it in your urethra.

If you have these symptoms and you have not been tested for menopause I suggest that you do. It is a blood test to check for certain levels of hormones to indicate if you are menopausal or post-menopausal, and if you are, then HRT could be part of the solution to solve this type of cystitis. You may also consider regular acupuncture.

## Type 17: Bladder Cancer

Like anywhere in the body, cancer cells can be in the bladder. I imagine this is excruciating and I hope sufferers have a good support system in place.

No matter what stage the cancer is, it is wise not to despair. It may be dealt with medical procedures and some protocols. It may be necessary in extreme cases to have the bladder surgically removed. Whatever the situation, a positive attitude and holistic as well as medical approach may increase the chances of recovery.

A positive attitude and self-talk could make a massive difference.

It is very hard to identify cancer of the bladder on your own, as the symptoms are also the same for other types of cystitis. Possible symptoms are: needing to pee frequently, even if there is no urine there; blood in the urine; pain or burning when peeing; flu-like symptoms, fever, and frequent urinary tract infections.

If you suffer frequently with UTIs it is crucial to get a camera in your bladder. This procedure is a cystoscopy. They numb your urethra with a gel, or other types of anaesthetic, then insert a tiny camera on a tube, called a cystoscope, up the urethra into the bladder. They usually fill up the bladder with water, also passed through the tube to inflate it so they can have a proper look at the walls.

You will need to be referred to a urologist, (urinary tract medical specialist).

If it is cancer you will most likely also be seen by a clinical oncologist, a cancer expert dealing with chemotherapy and radiotherapy, and/or a pathologist, an expert in diseased tissue.

It is important to get treatment as soon as possible. If a tumour is still small, it may not have spread to your muscles or out of your bladder, and so it may be easier to eradicate. Sometimes this can be done under general anaesthetic with a cystoscopy, cutting away the tumours, sealing the lining, and perhaps leave you with a catheter for few days to help drain the bladder of blood or urine.

Once it has spread, it is harder to treat, involving further treatments and medication. Chemotherapy may be applied directly into the bladder with a catheter if required.

If the damage is extensive it may be best to remove the bladder, this is a cystectomy. Surgeons will arrange an alternative way to evacuate the urine from your body, which is a procedure called urinary diversion.

## The Causes

It can be hereditary of course, but in most cases, cancer is due to personal lifestyle of sorts or past lifestyle catching up. The healthier the lifestyle, the fewer the risks, although there are exceptions. Sometimes there doesn't seem to be a logical or medical reason at all why cancer strikes, but there will be a hidden or metaphysical reason as I don't believe in coincidences. Some linked causes to bladder cancer are smoking, radiation, untreated viruses, leucoplakia, exposure to carcinogens, obesity, hormone problems, chronic inflammation, poor lifestyles and frequent UTIs.

If you are on your body's side, living in a harmonious way, such as excellent diet, great hydration, exercise within your limitations, plenty of fresh air, no alcohol, no smoking, no drugs, following the protocols and have a positive outlook, then you are doing all you can for your health and are less likely to get cancer.

Bladder cancer has links to smoking. Smokers are approximately four times more likely to get bladder cancer than non-smokers.

We all know people who drink, smoke, don't get much sleep, have poor hygiene, or sleep around without protection and yet are healthy and never had bladder issues or cancer. Good for them, but remember they are the exception, not the norm, so why not do all we can to avoid ill health and a cancerous future?

Cancer is not a foreign body or an infection, it is a mutated cell. It is a collection of confused genes that are receiving the wrong signal and duplicating malformed and too fast. They have gone rogue.

Smoking is linked to bladder cancer as the chemicals in cigarettes or any tobacco products, are highly carcinogenic – cancer-causing.

Other chemicals also play a part in cancer-forming and not just cancer but ill health in general: certain dyes, paints, petroleum, gases, plastics, rubbers, and asbestos.

The following are particularly toxic, although most of these are now banned they were used in the past in various industries and products: aniline dyes; naphthylamine; aminobiphenyl; xenylamine; benzidine; o-toluidine.

Even though nowadays exposure to certain chemicals in the workplace is minimal, cancer from exposure in a certain industry could take decades to manifest.

So, if you have had a job in an industry that deals with any of the chemicals above, and you suffer from bladder issues, do mention this to your doctor and get the tests necessary to check for cancer and other bladder ills.

Sometimes what cures us makes us ill in other areas. Chemotherapy and radiotherapy are harsh chemicals, so what you sometimes need to treat cancer is also cancer-forming. If you had these treatments for cancer somewhere else in your body, it could contribute to causing bladder cancer.

Bladder issues and cancer are linked to diabetes. So, do what you can to treat diabetes and have proper health-promoting nutrition, to avoid diabetes issues affecting your bladder.

If you have needed a long-term catheter, an indwelling, due to nerve damage or paralysation, this could also affect your bladder with infections, and potentially cancer.

If you have a weakened bladder due to long term or frequent UTI's, bladder infections, this could lead to bladder cancer, which is why it is important to be properly treated for every UTI.

If you have had bladder stones for a long period of time, this could irritate the lining and promote cancer.

Early menopause could also be linked to bladder cancer. Get diagnosed as soon as possible if you are having menopausal symptoms, even if you are considered too young. I started my menopause by 37 but was not diagnosed until 41, after they tested me for other stuff such as diabetes, thyroid and clinical depression.

When nothing else worked they checked my hormones and discovered I had been menopausal for some time, years in fact.

There is a certain infection, schistosomiasis, caused by parasites in water that if not treated properly, could be linked to bladder cancer.

Ensure all infections are properly treated and monitored. Please be mindful of where you swim or bathe, remember all parasites, bacteria, viruses, pollutants or toxins that live in water, can travel up your urethra and settle in your bladder.

Please tell your loved ones, colleagues, and friends if you have bladder cancer. Explain how it makes you feel, and ask for the help you need.

*No more taboos. No more hiding. The bladder needs airing.*

## Type 18: Prolapsed Bladder/Cystoceles/Fallen Bladder

This is a mechanical issue, not an internal bladder issue such as wall-lining defects or infection. The bladder is usually supported by the front wall of the vagina. When the bladder is empty it is obviously less heavy and more compact. When it fills up with urine it gets heavier. An average wee is approximately 600mls, but certain larger bladders can hold up to 1.5 litres when trained to keep it in ( I know as I could hold that much). A really large and full bladder could then weigh up to approximately 2 kilos, although on average it is *much* less and when empty it weighs whatever your organ size is. It is important not to train yourself to hold on but to have a wee often, keeping the bladder light.

If the vaginal wall gets weak, then it gives way and no longer fully supports the bladder. This can happen because of childbirth, vaginal surgery, womb problems affecting the vagina, or deterioration with age. Like leaning against a wall in a squat position and you go a bit too far and slide down.

When this happens, the bladder dislodges itself a little bit and it sinks. It is no longer fully supported, so it is pressured to hold itself within you, and at this point, you may notice you cannot hold onto as much urine as before.

Other symptoms may appear such as incontinence, peeing yourself, especially when you laugh, cough, sneeze or trip, difficulty peeing and a painful bladder or sensation of something needing to evacuate, like when you need a poo but can't go, a similar sensation in your lower abdomen, where your bladder is no longer where it needs to be and collapsing into the top of your vaginal area.

There are different grades of prolapse depending on the position of the bladder.

Grade 1 is mild, so only a small part of the bladder is sinking into the vaginal area.

Grade 2 is medium, where the bladder reaches the opening of the vagina.

Grade 3 is severe, where the bladder sticks out of the body and through your vagina.

Grade 4 is critical, where the entire bladder is out of your body through your vagina. This is very serious. At this stage, you could suffer from other prolapsed organs such as uterine, your womb collapsing, or rectocele, your rectum prolapsing.

Prolapse of the bladder is also linked with menopause because we produce less oestrogen. This hormone helps, among so many things, to keep the muscles around the vaginal area powerful, so this a great reason to take HRT if you are prematurely menopausal.

Usually, the menopause is around 50 years old. Getting it before 40 is considered premature and at that age, your body really does still need oestrogen production. This hormone is not just for bladder and pelvic muscles strength, but for bone density and other crucial things.

If you have premature or early menopause, do seek professional and holistic help.

**Probable causes of prolapse**

Childbirth, lifting heavy objects, forcing too much on the toilet, coughing for too long, constipation, any trauma to the pelvic or coccyx area, menopause.

Symptoms of prolapse can be like cystitis, but also feeling a lump in your vagina that isn't usually there. There could be extra pain in the pelvic area, a sensation that you haven't fully emptied your bladder after going for a wee, leaking urine, even more, frequent UTI's, really painful sex, lower back pain, difficulty in pooing.

Depending on the grade of the prolapse, you may hardly feel anything at all, or be in agony as you give birth to your own bladder.

Seek medical help if you believe you have this disorder. The treatment will depend on the grade. There are pessaries, a small device to hold the bladder in place, creams, HRT to replace oestrogen production, there are certain strengthening exercises, there is also surgery if need be. To help strengthen your pelvic floor, there are certain exercises to do and yoga or Pilates may also help. It is imperative to check with your medical team about exercise or other treatments if you have any stage of prolapse.

Seek medical help and gather all your options. Increase your own power by knowing what you can do for yourself, and also get the help of holistic therapists, or whom I like to call 'functional practitioners'.

Find out any personal energy links to your bladder such as abuse or abandonment.

Remember linguistic clues. Where do you feel you *have let yourself down*? Have *fallen through the gaps*/been ignored? Have *let yourself go*, or have *been misplaced or re-homed negatively*, where have you *lost your way*?

## Type 19: Malformed Bladder

This is a mechanical issue, where the bladder or urinary tract system defected during formation in the womb. It was not formed properly, this could be the bladder itself, the lining or problems with the tubes or the sphincter. Remember visualising the bladder as a bagpipe. Imagine some of the pipes not fitting right, then the air would leak out. If the stitching on the bag was not done right and letting out air, the whole system would not work properly.

It is not common to have a malformed bladder but it exists and there are surgeries to help fix it. Usually, malformation of the bladder means there are likely to be other formation issues, such as spina bifida.

If, as a baby, you had surgery for a defected urinary tract it may have left that area weak and prone to cystitis or prolapse.

Following the protocols will increase your chances of strengthening your waterworks.

## Type 20: Neurogenic Bladder

This is a specific issue due to a nerve problem, either temporary or permanent. If you had an accident or trauma that rendered you paraplegic or damaged your spinal cord, then your bladder could suffer.

It could be temporary, such as damaged coccyx. I went down a very high and fast waterslide recently and hit the water with too much force on my coccyx and butt and this damaged it enough to alter the nerve signals to the bladder. As a result, whilst my coccyx area was healing from the inflammation, I had mild but constant cystitis and urethritis. It lasted for 6 months, then the urethra and bladder slowly went back to normal but the coccyx still really hurt and sent spasms when I got up or sat down. I'm lucky that the impact didn't also displace my bladder or womb.

For me, the temporary neuro cystitis was more of discomfort in the urethra and the whole pelvic area rather than painful. What helped ease it was warm baths with pink salt, acupuncture and abiding by the protocols. The coccyx itself, however, was really painful.

It can be permanent if you damage the spinal column anywhere. Damaged or severed nerves are seriously problematic.

This is a bladder dysfunction, flaccid or spastic, caused by neurologic damage. Symptoms can be like cystitis, including overflow incontinence, the urgency to wee, need to wee frequently, or retention, so not weeing at all.

This is important to treat, as the risk of infection or vesicoureteral reflux or autonomic dysreflexia is high.

Medics will find a way to release the urine, to trigger urination.

Common issues that may cause this type of bladder problem are trauma to the spine or nerves, stroke, meningomyelocele, diabetes, alcoholism, severe vitamin B12 deficiency, herniated disks, pelvic injury, Parkinson's, multiple sclerosis, syphilis.

In a flaccid neurogenic bladder, the volume of urine is high but the pressure is low and contractions are not happening.
In men, this can also come with erectile dysfunction.

In a spastic bladder, the volume is normal or small and involuntary contractions are present.

It is possible to get both flaccid and spastic bladders at the same time or one followed by the other.

There are various ways to treat this, depending on the severity and cause. Medical solutions could involve: catheterisation, the use of short term or long term catheters; medication, there are several depending on the types of issue and other factors in personal health; surgery, could be a simple operation to insert a mechanical sphincter, or if really bad, remove the bladder altogether and introduce drainage alternatives.

There are a lot of metaphysical issues and trapped emotions associated with long-term bladder problems, which also need addressing on the journey to happy bladder health.

More on that later, but do start thinking about impacts your physical bladder issues have had on your mental, emotional, spiritual and social levels.

*Post in the Facebook tribe if you need support or advice or if you are going through this and can offer support to others, see community protocols.*

## Type 21: Bladder Stones

A common place to get stones is in the kidneys, but we can also have them in the bladder. These are balls of minerals and calcium that form in the bladder.

This happens when minerals, salts in concentrated urine, so dehydrated wee, crystalline and solidify into stones. It happens when you don't empty your bladder properly, so old wee nestles on the wall, calcifying and hardening.

Prostate gland enlargement in men can cause bladder stones and also damaged nerves, so a neurogenic bladder can contribute to these.

Inflammation of the bladder can also contribute to stones, as can radiation therapy anywhere in the pelvic area, catheters especially long-term, and if you have kidney stones, even though they are not the same, but if small enough to pass into your bladder and settle rather than get peed out, these can grow larger and become bladder stones.

Symptoms are like common cystitis but will also include acute abdominal pain and blood in the urine. If the stones are near the sphincter then they could also cause an obstruction and therefore block some of the urine inside the bladder and create some incontinence.

You may pass the stones naturally in your urine if they are small enough, but you may need medication to dissolve them, or surgery to remove them. Of course, the following will also help: working out what lead to forming these stones; changing any diet contributors; keeping well hydrated at all times; and taking your time to evacuate your wee properly.

It is important to tell your doctor about any urinary tract issue: do not live with it.

Early diagnosis of any bladder issue may avoid bladder stones or further damage and suffering. Drink plenty of clean water, between 1.5 and 5 litres per day depending on your size, to help flush out the stones. Get medical advice on this if you are unsure how much you should drink.

### Type 22: Urethral Syndrome/Symptomatic Abacterriuria/ Non-Specific Urethritis (NSU). Urethral Stenosis/Stricture

The same things that can affect the bladder can also irritate the urethra. It may be that you do not have bladder issue but the burning and strange sensation you are feeling is only in the urethra.

There are several causes such as dirty sex, STDs, bacterial, viral, menopausal dryness, neuro/nerves, where you trapped a nerve or the signal to that area is damaged due to trauma or impact to the spine or coccyx (this can include from spanking, again no judgement, just saying).

When there seems to be no explanation for this and there is no infection, then it is classed as non-specific. The urethra is just inflamed for some reason. I class this as either metaphysical, candida or unknown.

Following the protocols will help. Also drinking aloe vera may help. If it is due to dryness then you can use pessaries of oestrogen to be inserted into your vagina and this will help to lubricate the vaginal walls and penetrate the urethra too.

Most of the time urethritis will go away on its own within three months, however, do still get it checked by a doctor to look for infection. This is usually identified by having your pee analysed and your urethra swabbed with a cotton-bud.

If it is due to nerve damage or trauma of sorts, your doctor may suggest medication to help appease the nerves or inflammation such as ibuprofen, amitriptyline or gabapentin, however please note that I had severe reactions to these and had to come off them, so ensure, as with any medication, that you are followed regularly by a doctor and that you take note of any symptoms or reactions.

It is also important not to come off them instantly but to gradually wean off these drugs, again under medical advisement.

## Type 23: Chemically Induced

Some chemicals (man-made and organic) are linked to urinary issues and bladder cancer.

If you have worked in an industry where you have been exposed regularly to the following, then that could be the cause of your urinary symptoms and potential bladder cancer.

Aniline dyes, naphthylamine, aminobiphenyl, xenylamine, o-toluidine.

Aromatic amines, benzidine, beta-naphthylamine, pesticides, carcinogen benzene

Coal

Aluminium

Arsenic

Asbestos

Formaldehyde

Some Anti-Cancer Drugs such as cyclophosphamide

Chemotherapy, Radiotherapy, X-Rays, Nuclear Energy

Cigarettes/Cigars/Pipe smoking

Diesel Exhaust Fumes

OK, so we may be in contact with some of these chemicals without knowing it, so here is a list of industries where you may be exposed to them:

Manufacturing dyes, leather, rubber, aluminium, textiles, paints, nail varnishes, cigarettes.

Coal miners, tar-pavers, painters, hairdressers (who deal a lot with dyes), beauticians who do lots of manicures/pedicures.

Chemicals in food and additives can also be an irritant to the urinary tract and linked to bladder cancer. Among these are sweeteners, sugars and using a microwave, cooking meat over an open flame and using silicone or non-stick pans.

Chemicals found in daily products for cleaning and body-care can also irritate the urinary tract.

Following the nutritional protocols (we explore those soon) will help not consume chemicals from food, drink and cooking.

The medical protocols should help with not having unnecessary medications and talking to your doctor about drug side-effects.

The products protocol will help select the best products for your skin and home.

Quit smoking, seriously, the chemicals in cigarettes are linked to bladder cancer, and your smoke exhalations cause irritation to others, called passive-smoking.

Take precautions where possible such as covering your nose and mouth when dealing with petrol, diesel, nail varnish, perfumes.

If you are currently working in any of the industries linked to the bladder or other cancers, seriously evaluate your situation and taking precautions, or consider changing jobs.

### Type 24: Schistosomiasis/Snail Fever/Bilharzia

A disease caused by flatworm parasites that infect the urinary system and intestines. This is mainly caught by drinking or swimming in infected water. You will need medical assistance to clear them in the form of anti-worming medication. Be aware the worms live inside the blood vessels of your bladder, but their eggs can be peed out, so look out for eggs in our urine as a sign. Severe bloating of the abdomen can also be a sign.

### Type 25: Other Ills Linked to Cystitis or Precious Holes

We will explore these in the next chapter.

### Potential Cystitis Triggers for ALL of the 25 types

Just a reminder here of what can trigger any cystitis, because we know, don't we, that repetition is crucial. Bear in mind I mean *all* cystitis types, not just a UTI. Sometimes we just get a weird feeling and it goes away after we drink water, other times it is worse, so not all these will trigger an infection. You may only ever have had a few of these, depending on the most common type you suffer from. Being aware of all the potential triggers will help you understand how to avoid getting several types of cystitis too.

*As you read through them, tick the ones that you know triggered a cystitis type for you. This will help the information sink in. Remember we are a team, and this is a conversation, not just me talking, so please get involved.*

**The most common triggers are dehydration, alcohol and dirty sex.**

- Dehydration

We need water to make water, and we need water to make urine. The more water we have extra for the kidneys to trap the toxins in the better. Think of it like a glass of orange squash. If you put half a glass of neat squash in half glass water, it will be undrinkable, very intense. If you put a teaspoon of squash in a glass of water, it will be hardly noticeable, and this is what we want for our bladder.

Urine will sit in the bladder for a while, so it is important that it is as diluted as much as possible, so that fewer toxins or bacteria get to touch the walls.

The second reason why it is important to drink plenty of water is to wee more frequently, that way the same urine doesn't sit for too long in the bladder.

Good hydration lubricates the tubes and the wall lining. The moister the better, as dryness could end up cracking the skin and trapping germs.

The body needs water and that's the only fluid it truly needs. In my opinion, any other drink does not count towards your water intake. Some fluid will take away from your water, which means if you drink a cup of coffee or alcohol, then instead of adding one cup of fluid towards your allowance, you are taking one away.

**Some doctors, therapists or nutritionists say that all fluids count towards your water intake and that all fluids hydrate, but I certainly disagree.**

Would you put paint or coffee in your car and say that all fluids are the same, they all count? Of course not. Cars are designed to run on petrol or diesel. Humans are designed to run on proper food and water. Water, not *any* fluid.

- Malnutrition: eating the wrong foods and drinks, especially sugars, sweeteners, gluten, dairy, alcohols, caffeine, chemicals, pesticides.

- Sex/masturbation.

- Menopause. Hormone Fluctuations.

- Weight gain/Being Obese

- All bad hygiene habits including poor toilet, daily washing or sexual.

- Rushing your toilet time, pushing too hard or too fast.

- Holding on too long to your wee: this could be a problem, not only because you may pee yourself in public, but also because old wee will impregnate the bladder walls, and if your bladder and ureters are full, then your kidneys will have nowhere to send the toxic urine and may get infected and blocked. A full bladder will weigh more and could lead to prolapse if you do it often. You are also ignoring the nerve signals telling you to empty which may result in you becoming insensitive to them in the future, and may contribute to nerve issues in that area. So, please, pee when you need to.

- Clothing: anything touching your precious holes will be a trigger, especially tight trousers, tights, or the wrong underwear. This causes too much heat, chaffing, no air circulation, trapping germs.

- Products: anything you put on your skin will go inside your body. Simple. Be mindful of products you use. Read labels. Beware of what is in your soap, shampoo, conditioner, hair dye, toothpaste, mouthwash, moisturiser, deodorant, make-up, perfume, nail varnish, room-sprays, cleaning house products, polish, washing up liquid, washing powder, fabric softener, lubricants, and what your partner uses on their skin before touching you.

- Medication: including supposed health drinks, sports drinks, energy powders or manufactured smoothies, cranberry juice, cystitis sachets, prescribed medication and recreational drugs.

- Tobacco: smoke gets in the lungs, on your fingers, and in your blood and bladder. Smokers are 4 times more likely to get bladder cancer.

- Polluted water: drinking it or bathing in it. If water has bacteria in it, and you drink it or bathe in it, it may end up in your digestive system, and your urinary tract. Be mindful of the quality of water you use to wash with, drink, or brush your teeth with. It all counts.

- Thrush/Candida/Infections/Diarrhoea/Infected Menstruation/Leucoplakia: anything coming from any of your precious holes can cross-infect one another.

- Tampons/Sanitary towels

- Alcohol/Sugars/Dairy/Sweeteners/Caffeine/Chemicals/Gluten

- Reaction to certain medications

- Viruses including Epstein-Barr EBV

- Bacteria such as Streptococcus and E.Coli

- Metaphysical imbalances and blocked energies

- Stress

- Prostate Issues

- Sexually transmitted diseases

- Surgery, especially anywhere in the pelvic area

- Medical procedures such as smear tests, colposcopy, camera in the bladder or womb or colon and any numbing gels used

- Exposure to certain chemicals

- Shock: can also affect your adrenal glands and your womb, producing adrenal fatigue and random periods.

- Fear or anxiety

- Poor lifestyle choices

- Smoking or taking drugs

- Lack of sleep

- Lack of self-awareness or self-love

- Issues with red or orange chakras and imbalances in the aura

- Getting too cold or staying in damp clothing

- Self-fulfilling belief patterns: thinking you will get cystitis may bring it on as thoughts become reality, so be aware of your self-talk.

- Using cystitis as an excuse, saying you have it when you don't, hence wishing it on yourself.

- Depression

- Victimisation/Bullying

- Rape or abuse

- Saying yes when you wanted to say NO

- Inauthenticity or lying about having cystitis= self-fulfilling prophecy

- Poverty or poverty belief pattern/Destitution

- Using commercial or toxic products to wash or do laundry with

- Using bath-bombs or bubble bath

- Wearing tight knickers/throngs/G-strings/tight trousers or lycra

- Getting cold, walking barefoot on cold tiles, staying in damp clothes

- Trauma to the coccyx

- Spinal or nerves injury

- Catheters

- Other bladder issues

- Pregnancy

- Abnormal lumps in the pelvic area

- Childbirth

- Urinary Incontinence (UUI, SUI, Overflow, Functional and Bedwetting)

- Bladder Cancer

- Kidney Cancer or Kidney disease

- Fibromyalgia/Chronic Fatigue/Autoimmune Diseases/ Diabetes/Dementia

- Female Genital Mutilation or Circumcision

- Metaphysical blockages or imbalances

* * *

## Chapter 4 Keynotes

- There are 25 types of/main causes of cystitis.

- Knowledge is key. Knowing about cystitis 'triggers' will help us avoid them.

- Words have power: be mindful of your self-talk or how you allow others to talk to you.

- All the levels of life, so physical, mental, emotional, sexual, spiritual, social, and environmental, will affect our bladder.

- Sex is a huge contributor to cystitis in many ways.

- Bladders are a simple design (a bag for holding fluid) but can be affected by many issues, most of which are treatable and avoidable.

- Claim back your power and be in charge of your bladder.

- Cystitis means inflammation of the bladder, but there are other bladder problems that are not officially classed as cystitis, even though they give similar symptoms.

- It is imperative to get medical advice and tests done to check your bladder and kidneys if you suffer from *any* urinary tract issues.

- Following the protocols will help with all bladder issues. With UTIs, cancer, prolapse, or neuro bladder, there are necessary medical procedures and treatments to also consider.

## Action! Interactive bit, it's your turn:

1. What have you read in this chapter that really hit the spot? Have you found a nugget of gold yet? If so what is it and how can you apply it to your health?

2. In your journal mark down your food and drink and when you get any cystitis symptoms. Start identifying why you get the symptom and link it to a trigger. Knowledge is power. Claim it.

3. Write down all the types of cystitis you have already suffered from and their potential triggers.

4. Right now, compliment yourself. That's right, start practising healthy self-talk. Write down 7 new healthy mantras in your journal and repeat them daily.

Here are a few examples to start you off:

'I am amazing just for being me.'

'I am proud that I am learning about bladder health, as I am powerful and in control of my life quality.'

'I am beautiful, happy, and all is well.'

'I totally rock!'

So, now that we have delved into 24 different types of cystitis, I hope you are starting to understand how knowledge is power. By the end of this book, you will have all the necessary tools to change your bladder health and your life.

So we continue on our technical stretch of the journey.

Let's take a closer look at cystitis type 25 now…

# Other Ills Affecting the Bladder & Precious Holes. Cystitis Type 25.

This book is about different types of cystitis, which means inflamed bladder, but there are other issues that I classed under *cystitis type 25*.

We need to acknowledge these in detail, so this chapter is about those.

All protocols will help any bladder or urinary issue, even a healthy bladder to be healthier and remain fully functioning for a long lifetime.

Don't worry we get into those in the next chapter. We are building up momentum and a good knowledge base first.

So, if you suffer from any other illness or condition, be sure to still read the entire book and implement all the protocols possible.

Any other bladder ailment will weaken the area and so be prone to cystitis.

Use this book as a preventative, not just for potential healing.

**Let us explore other reasons why the bladder may be unhappy :o(**

## Urgency Urinary Incontinence/Overactive OAB

This is more a symptom of other bladder issues, but sometimes can stand alone, so I have classed this in the main cystitis section also but will repeat it here.

This is where you cannot hold your pee very well and you leak. This happens when muscles are too weak and cannot control urine leaking out of the sphincter. The plug is not quite doing its job and so any stress on the area will push wee out.

It can also happen if your bladder muscles are too active. This is an overactive bladder where it is too enthusiastic, giving you the signal you urgently need a wee, but you don't. This is different from cystitis when you need to pee but nothing is there. This type is sometimes called 'urge incontinence'.

It can also be linked to diabetes that is untreated, called 'polyuria', where too much urine is produced.

This bladder malfunction can also be classed as the irritable bladder, but I have decided to give that its own section under a type of cystitis, IBS, for it is so common and not easily diagnosed or even discussed.

The remedies vary from pelvic exercises to medication or devices. There are plenty of functional remedies that could help including working on the emotional and social impact incontinence creates, to ensure the ripple effect doesn't become a tsunami.

## Diabetes

Polyuria is a symptom of diabetes when too much urine is produced and that affects the bladder and can contribute to urine urgency.

Due to sugar issues within the system caused by diabetes, this leaves the bladder more prone to cystitis, as we know sugar feeds candida and irritates bladder walls. What I recommend is to ensure that if you do have diabetes, that you research what to do to fully be in control of it, including a great diet, plenty of water, and to be on top of any medication.

Ensure you are followed regularly by your doctor or medical professional to understand diabetes and how to help yourself. The more you are aware of how to deal with this disease, the less it will affect your bladder health. Remember that sugar is the bad guy for both diabetes and candida cystitis, so be mindful of what you eat.

## Fibromyalgia and Chronic Fatigue

Pain in the body or being exhausted most of the time. It can be worsened by hormone imbalances, periods, menopause, stress, depression, fatigue and bladder issues.

IC, so chronic cystitis can accompany fibromyalgia, as it can affect the nervous system, and so can be linked to neuro-bladder symptoms.

Vice versa, the constant chronic pain and irritation from having IC could lead to the nerve issues linked to fibromyalgia and ME/chronic fatigue. This is also known as central sensitization when the nervous system (nerves) is associated with developing and maintaining chronic pain.

Whatever you can do to alleviate fibromyalgia or chronic fatigue will help you not also get chronic cystitis.

Some say taking antihistamines to keep allergies under control helps with IC, and so is ensuring to avoid foods that irritate or inflame.

## Dementia/Alzheimers

UTIs symptoms may differ somewhat with older people suffering from dementia issues. It is imperative to look out for increased signs of confusion, agitation, withdrawal, and delusions, as these may be signs of an untreated bladder infection. As we know, untreated infections can lead to sepsis or bladder cancer.

UTIs can intensify dementia symptoms and can also speed up the progression of dementia.

## Menopause

I have indeed mentioned this under the *Menopausal Cystitis*, but it is such a huge subject that affects women's health that I wanted to elaborate here.

Hormone fluctuations play a huge role in a woman's life. We start around age 10 to 13 with preparation for childbearing and start our periods, also known as menstruation. This is when we become fertile and an egg is released monthly for fertilisation. If it isn't fertilised then the lining of the womb sheds and we bleed.

Personally, I find this a really crappy system, especially for those of us who decide or who are unable to have children, then we suffer from periods for decades, literally for NOTHING. If I would have known as a teenager or young adult that I would not have children I would have considered removing the womb. The ovaries can still produce the hormones necessary but as far as I'm aware the womb really only exists as a home for a baby to grow, and menstruation as part of that cycle. I don't recommend this (womb removal) to anyone, as hindsight is both a blessing and a curse, and we can't know if we will want children or not in the future, so I'm just venting! Although when I was bleeding three times a month for months and became anaemic, some friends told me they had their wombs removed and it was life-changing and liberating. Luckily the medics found out I was having a reaction to a certain HRT patch and I came off them and the problem stopped.

So if you have womb issues, make sure you find a good doctor and specialist to discuss your options.

When we start running out of eggs (we are born with all our eggs in our ovaries already) our body prepares for the post-fertility stage. We produce less oestrogen and we go through a big change.

Some women go through this and barely notice, others feel it a lot.

I felt it a lot. I had premature menopause by age 37 and went undiagnosed for two years as the symptoms were similar to depression. So if you suffer, ask your doctor to do a blood test to check for your levels of FSH, LH, Oestradiol, and Iron.

In case it helps you identify it, my menopause symptoms were:

- Dry flaky skin especially on arms and shins
- Papery skin on my hands, like fast ageing
- Increased and darker facial hair
- Irregular and heavier periods
- Mood swings
- Not feeling myself/being tetchy
- Fainting
- Nausea
- Depression
- Rapid weight gain, especially around the midriff
- Hot flushes, especially during the night
- Exhaustion

- Cystitis and irritable urethra
- Forgetfulness
- Lack of drive or passion
- Spoonerism – mixing up the first letters of two words, for example, The Red Table would be the Ted Rable. Or in sentences too, as I once said:

*'Oh, crap. I've pissed the most again.'*

I looked at Mum who was smirking and I knew I'd said something wrong again. By then she was used to it and replied 'it's OK, I know what you meant.'

And of course what I meant was:

*'Oh, crap. I've missed the post again.'*

Although in some cases it was funny, especially as the humour was unintentional, it did get on my nerves after a while. Luckily this went away once I was on HRT. I'm not saying this is a symptom of menopause as it may have been a reaction to the mix of medication I was on at the time for depression, anxiety, trauma and stress, but it's still worth mentioning.

The menopause happens usually around age 50 to 55 years and if you go through it then, the symptoms may be less as the body is no longer designed to have the same hormone levels.

If however, you have the menopause earlier, then it can be problematic.

For premature I suggest having HRT patches because the body still needs these hormones for bone density, mood regulation, skin elasticity and lubrication, although make sure you talk to your doctor about the risks involved and all of your options.

It is far too early to have the menopause before age 40. Find a type of HRT that suits you. The one with different doses suited me, but when I moved onto the continuous patch, I bled every 8 days and it did not suit me. Find a good doctor to help you through your options.

So here are some suggestions that may alleviate symptoms, they helped me:

- HRT Patches (under doctor's advisement and with 6 monthly reviews, ensure you get the type that suits you).
- High-quality Aloe Vera Gel drink
- Acupuncture
- Exercise/Movement, especially outside in nature
- Regular Meditations
- Good quality supplements of Omega 3, vitamin C, iron, vitamin D3, Calcium, zinc, magnesium and vitamin B12
- Great nutrition (following the nutrition protocol and anti-candida regime may help.)
- I also went on antidepressants for a couple of years at the start, as I was also clinically depressed. I don't recommend medication unless it's necessary so really talk to your doctor and tune into your body.

**Caution**: I tried three types of antidepressants before finding the one that suited me. The only one that worked for me was a drug called *citalopram*. As with all medication follow your doctor's advice. The other two medications made things a lot worse and I had to come off them. I read the side-effects of one type and it warned that taking it could bring on suicidal thoughts and acts of violence! WTF. Let's invent a drug to help those patients who are severely depressed and barely clinging to life, and it will either work or push them over the edge.

Only take medication prescribed by a doctor that you trust. If on antidepressants and HRT make sure you are followed up regularly and keeping notes of your symptoms.

Do not come off medication suddenly. Both antidepressants and HRT mess with your hormones and brain chemicals of sorts, and you absolutely need to follow your doctor's orders on how to take them, for how long, and how to come off them.

If you are on any kind of medication, keep a journal to track any changes, improvements or issues. Sometimes we need medication, but being in tune with your body will help you know when it's time to ask your doctor to help you come off them.

Following the protocols will help keep the whole body fitter and healthier.

I found acupuncture was amazing to help reduce hot flushes and pain and enhance mood, and regulate bleeding.

Menopause isn't an illness or something that goes wrong, it is a healthy and normal part of womanhood, but it is part of women's issues that need addressing.

## Vaginal Dryness/Urethra Dryness

This is when the skin in your vagina and vulva (precious holes and flaps) or inside your urethra becomes thinner, less elastic and dry. The reason for this is mainly lack of oestrogen production, so post-menopause. Avoid commercial soaps and creams. Avoid chemicals such as bathing in swimming pools. Keep hydrated. Use a lubricant before sex, a good one not with nasties. Following the protocols is a good idea. And most of all, don't be embarrassed to ask for help or tell your partner. Unfortunately, about 60% of post-menopausal women suffer from painful dryness. This may also mean you have a dry urethra and therefore cause cystitis symptoms.

If you have this due to menopause but then put on weight with it, it may help, as excess fat also produces tiny amounts of oestrogen.

I didn't suffer from vaginal dryness but from urethra dryness. Even though I had premature menopause as I laid down so much tummy fat, my levels of oestrogen even without my eggs were not too bad due to being so overweight. I'm not saying that is a good thing as in general obesity is not good for health, however, we take the positives where we can, right?

And remember whatever our body does, it is to protect us, even though it may not feel like it. I put on weight for many reasons, one of them was due to lack of oestrogen at a young age, the body knew it still needed it to protect my bones, my organs and so much more, so it laid down fat *very* quickly to protect my ovaries and organs and also to help produce more oestrogen. Clever really.

Did I enjoy being obese going from a size 12 to 24 in 18 months? Oh, hell, no!

Am I angry at my body for it? Definitely not. The dude is just trying to keep me safe even during the duress of extreme hormone issues, due from menopause but also the contractive implant.

## Vaginal Thrush

Thrush in the vagina is common. It is also known as yeast or fungal infection or candida. This irritates not only the inside of your vagina but also the lips, so all your precious holes may be affected.

It is mainly caused by the imbalance in the gut microbiome, poor hygiene and diet.

Like cystitis, this is not a sexually transmitted disease but it can be brought on by 'dirty' sex. So, one way to ensure not getting it is to follow sexual and hygiene protocols.

Also, follow the anti-candida diet for a few weeks until cleared up and then be aware of your fulcrum, how much food from the no list you can tolerate. More on this later.

The following have been known to help me when I had vaginal thrush:

- Aloe Vera Gel drink
- Aloe Vera Gelly or cream on the vulva lips (I put this in the fridge so it is soothingly cold) and also insert some into the vagina
- Aloe Vera & Propolis Cream
- Anti-candida diet
- Plenty of fresh water
- Wearing no knickers or trousers
- Drink 1 tsp food-grade bicarbonate soda in water before bed
- Pessaries (to in the vagina, from a chemist or prescribed by a doctor)

Ensure to be hygienic and don't wipe any thrush over your urethra.

## Bacterial Vaginosis

This is similar to thrush, but it involves an infection in the vagina. It can be as a result of dirty sex, tampons, poor hygiene. See *Vaginal Thrush* as the treatment is similar.

This can be painful, itchy and produce a foul-smelling discharge.

Following the protocols will help avoid this. If you have it please, do get checked out by a doctor as antibiotics may be necessary.

## Bartholin's Blocked Glands/Vaginal Cysts

We have glands in our vagina that produce fluid, natural lubrication. At times these can get blocked and the trapped fluids form a cyst.

One way to get rid of those is to sit in hot baths (without any nasties in it, maybe salt or appropriate essential oils) to help it open up and drain.

A doctor can also drain it.

Sometimes antibiotics may be needed if it gets infected.

It may not cause cystitis but will affect your precious holes and so needs mentioning.

The idea is to keep your precious holes and flaps clean and healthy as if one is affected, the whole area may be.

## Lichen Sclerosus

Irritating patchy or thinning skin condition around the vulva (precious holes and flaps) these are usually non-cancerous. Menopause can also be linked to this condition.

To help treat this rub a high-quality aloe vera cream or a gel that you can tolerate on it and keep to the hygiene and sexual hygiene and hydration protocols.

Medically you may be offered steroid ointment. I would try natural alternatives first as steroids can thin the skin, and this condition is already doing that. You can have lichen anywhere on the body so be followed medically if you suspect you have this condition anywhere, as it may eventually lead to skin cancer over time, if not treated.

## Cervical Abnormal Cells/PAP/HPV

Having regular smear tests and colposcopies are recommended. They check for PAP which means cervical cell changes and HPV that denote infections.

Sometimes you will have abnormal cells reported.
Don't panic, this doesn't necessarily mean cancer, in fact in most cases it doesn't.

Medics use the term *pre-cancerous*. I don't think this is a good idea as in some people it could start a panic attack.

We either have cancer, or we don't.

Instead of pre-cancerous, they should just say no cancer detected but the result denotes that there is something not quite right and to keep it under supervision. I think another word needs to be used, as having the word *cancer* (pre-cancerous) makes us focus on cancer.

It is similar to saying as soon as you start your periods you become ***pre-pregnant***. The risk is there, the possibility and some conditions are promotive of pregnancy, but that does not mean you will get pregnant!

Cervix cells fluctuate and change as a woman goes through different stages.

Sometimes you get viruses and infections on the cervix that go way naturally, they usually sort themselves out. HPV is a sexually transmitted disease but one that most sexually active people will contract at some point and in most cases the body deals with it.

The only way to never get HPV is to never have sex, not even oral or anal, as this is transmitted skin to skin. As this is not likely, then the second-best way is to practice only safe/protected sex, so, using a condom and ensuring both partners are clean and do not have genital warts. It is also wise not to have any kind of sex with people who have had plenty of partners and who have practised unsafe sex.

There are HPV vaccines available, usually given to girls around 12 years old, and now given to boys too (in the UK) however just like any vaccine this does not ensure you will never get it, it just reduces the risks.

It also depends on your feelings on vaccinations, I'm not really a fan of any, but in such a medical and pressurised world, vaccinations are sometimes unavoidable.

Schools are now much better at sex education than they used to be (I didn't get any at my school in my era), however, it is important to really explain to children about sex, related diseases and pregnancy, to drum it in. If they are giving HPV vaccination to 12-year-olds, they also need to explain what it is, why they are getting it, and how to avoid all sexual diseases.

If they are old enough to have the injection, they are old enough to know everything related to sex and procreation.

The average age people start being sexually active seems to have dropped since my time at school, this is evident by the increase in teenage pregnancies.

HPV viral infections may go away on their own, however, it is best to keep being monitored, the norm is every six months, just to ensure they do not promote cancer.

If they do turn cancerous, there are many ways to be treated successfully.

Cervical cancer is also linked to smoking.

## Uterine Bleeding

We are used to having our menstruation. We bleed from our womb as a result of the lining shedding as we didn't fall pregnant that month. This is normal.

It sucks, but it's normal.

Sometimes, however, we bleed from the womb and it isn't a period. If you bleed outside of your menstruation time or are post-menopausal, it is important to be checked medically. There could be many reasons.

I was bleeding too much as a result of a reaction to a certain HRT patch, and other times due to a shock and emotional trauma and once because of a polyp.

Reasons for extra bleeds could be hormonal, thyroid problems, fibroids, polyps, cancer, infection, pregnancy, shock, trauma, miscarriage or pelvic inflammatory disease.

As well as a smear test or a colposcopy (that checks the vaginal canal and cervix) you may have to have a camera in the womb (hysteroscopy).

I know several women who had this done without anaesthetic or painkillers and were OK as it should feel like a smear test and then a slight period/menstruation pain whilst the camera passes into the womb.

This was not the case for me. I had been bleeding three times per months for over six months by the time I had my hysteroscopy and my cervix was so swollen that it needed a clamp to prise it open to pass the camera in. I needed the procedure a second time to remove a polyp and insisted on having it done in theatre under full anaesthesia.

## Linguistic interlude:

*Hysterika* is the Greek name for uterus/womb. It is where we get the word *hysteria* or *hysterical* from, as it was believed women were plagued by excessive emotion coming from the womb. More female anatomy being ridiculed!

The word *miscarriage* is unhealthy. It suggests the woman is to blame, as she did not carry the baby properly, which is not the case. There are many reasons why we lose babies and let's take the negative implication away from the word. Losing a baby is obviously very stressful and upsetting and we need to be checked out medically should we go through this.

* * *

## Pregnancy

OK, so being pregnant and giving birth are natural and not issues or ills, however, there are so many things that can go wrong during pregnancy or childbirth that it is worth mentioning in this section. I can't list them though as they are almost endless.

It is imperative that you do see a doctor once you know you are pregnant to ensure all is splendid.

And don't panic, there are many women that go through pregnancy and childbirth without complications, but in my family and circle of friends, it is not the case.

If you are pregnant and a cystitis sufferer, do ensure you look after your bladder and precious holes very well. Think positive thoughts, tell your body that it is safe and healthy and that all is well...

**Note:** we get the start of our microbiome, our gut flora from our mother's vagina as we are born, and then enhanced by breastfeeding.

If you have a cesarean (C-Section) you may wish to consider swabbing inside your vagina and smearing this on your baby on the day it is born, so that it mimics natural birth and getting what he needs from you. If you have an infection or bladder/uterine cancer at this time, do not do this.

## Folliculitis on the Groin/Thighs

Sometimes our hair follicles get blocked and swollen. When this happens on the groin or on your inner thighs it is really painful and irritating. They look like red boils and not usually squeezable, annoyingly. It is mainly swollen tissue.

What I found helps is:

- Dry skin brushing daily to keep skin smooth
- Cold showers
- Washing with only appropriate products
- There is also a wash/cream I have from the doctors that works well on this called Dermol Cream.

If they get infected you may need antibiotics as with any infection.

For any women's issues, please seek medical help.

## Chub-Rub

Cute name for the condition we get as our thighs rub together when walking.

When I was super slim (before hormone-related issues) I didn't suffer from this as my thighs didn't touch.

Since becoming 'voluptuous', I take the risk of setting my thighs on fire by walking too fast, another reason not to run, as spontaneous combustion is never a good look.

That said do not let being overweight or chub rub stop you running or exercising if you wish to, just take precautions for comfort such as wearing baggy cotton shorts long enough to cover your thighs, and wear a good support bra if needed, drink plenty of water and ensure good form and posture.

This is how I deal with Chub-Rub, aside from visualising slimmer thighs and an end to hormone issues:

- Wear cut off cotton pyjama bottoms under your skirts so that your thighs are covered, this provides a buffer zone whilst keeping your precious holes aired.
- Rub on cold aloe vera gelly (keep it in the fridge).
- Rub organic raw coconut oil on your thighs in the morning.
- Dry skin brushing daily to keep skin smooth.
- Drink high-quality aloe vera juice, because it helps most things.
- Do not use talcum powder or alcohol products. Talc is bad news for cystitis sufferers. It also clogs your skin, and it needs to breathe.

You will sweat and the talc will just become a gooey mess. If talc gets up the urethra and into the bladder it will cause much offence. Do not use talc on a nappy rash on babies either, again use the aloe cream or something similar. Let's respect all precious holes.

**Exception:** it is standard practice to have talc on the skin before any waxing. So when I have my Hollywood, I go to the loo straight after and have a wee to ensure any talc is pushed out the urethra. Then I use a wet flannel to touch-wipe the area, and then when I get home I have a cool shower with the aloe vera soap to ensure both wax and talc are properly removed.

**Flaps Flannel.** Yep, I may design a flannel just for cleaning our flaps, so watch this space. In the US, I believe the word for flannel is *facecloth*.

So ladies, get a facecloth just for your flaps.

*By now you are used to my unique vocab. Precious holes are inner labia, where the holes are. The flaps are outer labia, our bottom lips.*

**So basically, keep your precious holes and flaps clean at all times.**

## Diarrhoea

We can get the runs for many reasons: food poisoning, a virus, post-surgery, detoxing, medication, IBS and much more. The reason it gets mentioned here is because infected poo, the runny slippery kind, comes dangerously close to the vagina and urethra.

Be super-mindful to wipe front to back, wash and rinse properly after each bout.

Do not sit on the loo too long after diarrhoea as the germs could travel up into your open urethra. Wipe and flush then sit back down for more, if needed.

If symptoms persist seek medical assistance.

## Sexually Transmitted Diseases (STD)/Venereal Diseases (VD)

If you have any kind of unprotected sex you are hugely at risk of infecting your precious holes and where they lead to (bladder, cervix, womb, colon). Following sexual protocol will help you not get infections or thrush but will not prevent sexually transmitted diseases.

If you have unprotected sex (penis, fingers, vaginal, anal or oral) with someone who is not your long-term partner and that you not only trust to remain faithful but who has also had recent tests to check his or her sexual health, then you are at risk of diseases and pregnancy.

You can also catch some of these diseases through infected drug needles, passed from mother to infant during childbirth or breastfeeding, and blood transfusions.

**Sexually transmitted diseases include** chlamydia, gonorrhoea, chancroid, syphilis, crabs/pubic lice, genital herpes, Human Papillomavirus (HPV) which can lead genital warts and cancer, Human immunodeficiency (HIV)/Aids, hepatitis B, trichomoniasis, molluscum contagiosum.

Some diseases are not classed as STD's but can be passed on through sex or caused by it: cystitis, urethritis, UTI, thrush, meningitis, scabies, other infections or viruses, lice, skin rashes.

Seriously, that one night stand may not be worth it.

If your partner has cheated on you, then first off dump his sorry arse, then go to the doctors and ask to be screened (checked) for sexually transmitted diseases. It is free in the UK on the NHS and involves a smear test, blood tests and a urine test.

Condoms are cheap and easy to buy. They are also free on the NHS, just as contraceptive pills and other contraceptive methods, however, the pill will not save you from diseases, only from pregnancy, and it is not 100% effective.

If your non-trustworthy partner doesn't want to wear condoms then don't have sex with him. Apparently, there are plenty of decent men who would respect your sexual health and wear condoms and be clean before touching you.

**Stay away from the douchebags.**

I once asked my ex- GP, instead of giving me the contraceptive pill, could she give me a pill to stop me being attracted to douchebags? This was after screenings as my fiancée at the time turned out to be a sociopath and psychopath and already had another fiancée and two girlfriends (one of which a now ex-friend of mine) that I obviously didn't know about.

She laughed and said 'if only! The world is full of dirty bastards. No, there is no pill, the only way is to shoot them. Then she said, no, OK just avoid them.'

Avoiding all men forever is an option for sexual health and not having an unwanted pregnancy, but a tad extreme, so perhaps start with the condoms and being a bit pickier who you let touch you.

## Birth Control

This type could also fit under *sexual cystitis* or *medically induced* however I'm giving it its own entry here.

It is possible to get an infection (bladder or womb) or cystitis as a side effect or reaction from birth control pills or a coil, also known as an intrauterine device (IUD). If this happens you can ask for alternative birth control as there are many pills or patches and one may suit you more than another. Condoms are also an option.

**Important**: be aware that some contraceptive methods, especially the implant (a small device placed inside your arm and stays there for up to three years) can cause huge weight gain and of course, hormone imbalances.

I wasn't told this when my doctor at the time suggested I have it done as it was so convenient, she said. The irony is that the week I got it implanted I left my boyfriend as he was cheating on me, and devastated I stayed single, as in not even a kiss, for the next three years. What a total waste of time that implant was.

Within 18 months of having the implant, I had gained SO much weight, put it this way I went from a size 12 to a size 24.

I can't blame it all on the implant, I'm sure depression played a part, as did the premature menopause that came within that time-frame.

So due mainly to hormone issues (self-inflicted with the bloody implant and nature with menopause), I ballooned very quickly. For this reason, I do not recommend the implant or the pill. Condoms are the safest as far as I'm concerned because they prevent pregnancy and most sexually transmitted diseases. They don't stop those that are transferred from skin to skin contact as I assume you will cuddle naked and there will still be some penetration of sorts. Condoms can also break or rip.

Hindsight is a curse to us but a blessing to others, so just to say that if I knew then what I know now, I would NEVER have gone on the pill and never had that implant.

I would not have the coil either as I don't like the idea of a foreign object infiltrating my womb, however, I know some that are fine with them, and some that really are not. Discuss your options with your doctor, and tune into your body.

## Pelvic Inflammatory Disease (PID)

This is a bacterial infection in your pelvic area, usually stemming from germs from your vagina or cervix that move inward. A most common way to catch PID is through unprotected sex as chlamydia and gonorrhoea can lead to PID. You can also catch it without sex, for example, if you have an infection in your vagina, or anywhere on your precious holes and the bacteria spread up.

PID causes chronic pain anywhere in the lower abdomen, in some people it can be tolerable, in others agonising. You may also feel a weird sensation or pressure against your womb, fallopian tube area, so also your bladder.

So it is important if medically they have ruled out cystitis, to be checked for PID, as sometimes that weird sensation and pain we feel with cystitis, could be because we haven't really identified the right area (the womb/fallopian tubes, ovaries and bladder are very close). Untreated PID can result in infertility issues.

Following the protocols should help with not getting this.

## Piles/Colonic Polyps/Colorectal Cancer/Ulcerated Colitis/ Diverticulitis/IBS/Candida infestation in the bowels/Worms

There are many issues that can go wrong with our colon or bowels and if you suffer from any of these you may be more prone to cystitis or thrush and irritated precious holes. If your anus is itchy it may transfer to your vagina and urethra.

If you have any of these issues or have any pain, inflammation, blood or worms coming out of your anus or in your poo, you must seek medical help. The better you look after your bowels and anus, the better your bladder and womb will be too.

Remember that treating one precious hole well, and where it leads to, will help all the others. The body is connected and so if you follow the protocols in this book, that were predominantly written for bladder and urethra health, it will probably have a positive effect on the rest of your systems too.

Remember any *–itis* issue should be helped by following an anti-inflammatory diet, and drinking a high-quality aloe vera gel daily (start with a low dose of 30ml then increase to 100mls as it can be a diuretic and so can lead to diarrhoea when you are not used to it).

Not straining on the loo, proper hydration and using a *Squatty Potty* will also help to evacuate the bowels properly.

If your parents or grandparents had colon cancer, it may be wise to be checked at regular intervals to ensure all is well as it can be hereditary.

This involves having a smear of your poo analysed, or having a camera in the colon.

Speak to your doctor if you have any concerns.

They may refer you to a gastroenterologist, a doctor who specialises in problems with the digestive system including the intestines, or a proctologist, a doctor trained in problems with the rectum and anus.

If surgery is needed you will see a general surgeon.

## Specifically in men: Prostate & Scrotum Problems

As mentioned in the introduction, this book is written for my best girl, however, the information is useful for men too.

So this section is just for you, Dude, or for you my girl to pass onto a man in your life who suffers from any cystitis.

**Prostate:** the main link to bladder problems is the prostate. If you have recurring cystitis or urethritis, do get your prostate checked out.

If you have prostate issues, do have your urinary tract checked out.

Issues causing any type of cystitis or urethritis could be due to an enlarged prostate (benign prostatic hyperplasia/BPH), prostate cancer, kidney stones, any of the 25 cystitis types applicable to men, or an abnormal narrowing of the urethra, so a thinner pee/semen tube than normal.

**Scrotum:** it could also be due to issues with your scrotum such as epididymitis, testicular torsion, or a reaction in there resulting from abdominal problems including cystitis or kidney infection/disease.

**Erectile Dysfunction:** problems getting or sustaining an erection could also be linked to a type of cystitis, especially IC/BPS because it can cause inflammation leading to endothelial dysfunction, and then possibly ED.

Issues linked to cystitis also connected to ED are diabetes, hormone fluctuations, and kidney disease because they mess around with hormones levels, blood circulation and energy levels, and certain medications can also cause ED.

**Men and women have kidneys, ureters, bladders and urethras (Urinary Tract) and therefore the symptoms and pains of cystitis are the same.**

Homosexual men (so men who have sex with other men) are more likely to get UTI or candida cystitis than men who only have sex with women, however wearing condoms and following the sexual protocols should help reduce the risks.

**Extra things to look out for in men (although do read the entire book as it mostly does apply).**

- White or cloudy discharge from your precious hole, so the tip of your penis, also known as your *Bell-End :o)*

- Burning or weird sensation either from your bladder, your penis or your scrotum, when you pee

- Your Bell-End, so the tip of your penis is sore, bloody, swollen, irritated

- Problems getting it up (ED)

I repeat here because if you have read the entire book, Dude, you will know I like to repeat myself. Why? Well, because knowledge is key.

**So if you are a Dude, it is imperative you read the entire book and do the exercises that apply, obviously you cannot look in the mirror to explore your flaps, but for the most part, it applies to you too.**

## Female Genital Mutilation/Infibulation/Circumcision

Even though we live in the modern age of 2019, sadly in some countries girls and women are not only disrespected but disgustingly abused, and not only by men but other women too.

One of these ways is by female genital mutilation. Female circumcision using a blade usually performed soon after birth but some as late as puberty and adults too. This procedure 'ritual' can include removing the clitoral hood, clitoral glands, the inner labia and sometimes also cutting away not only the inner but also outer labia and then closing/sewing up the vulva. In this extreme ritual, called *infibulation*, a tiny hole is left for peeing and period and then when appropriate, the vagina can be opened for sex and childbirth.

**Note**: without the clitoral and receptors in the precious holes area and vaginal tunnel, no real sexual pleasure can be experienced, so sex really is for the male pleasure and reproduction only in this case, not to mention painful for the woman.

The health implications of these rituals are **endless**, not to mention constant cystitis and UTIs.

How the bloody hell is this still allowed?

Please let's show respect for the human body and nature, she knows best.

Disempowering girls and women in this misplaced belief to keep their virtue and to fit into a society where female parts are seen as dirty, slutty, unnecessary or impure, is truly damaging to them.

I love the diversity in all cultures, however, I can't get on board with this. It's beyond insane and barbaric and useless. It also causes so many health issues, and the emotional and mental issues are also endless.

The only way to truly stop cystitis issues from mutilation is to stop this ritual completely, making it illegal in *all* countries and enforcing this law.

At the moment it is banned in most countries, but not all, and not well monitored, so it does still go on.

If there is a true medical reason and performed by proper surgeons, then that is different. In boys and men, circumcision can be a good thing if it helps a man no longer be in pain due to a tight foreskin, and it also helps with hygiene as germs get trapped in the foreskin. Female mutilation is not the same thing and other than perhaps removing a cancerous lump on the labia, I can think of no good reason to cut any of it off.

Sadly if you have been through this female mutilation, first of all, I'm so sorry you were subjected to such inhumanity.

And second, please follow all the protocols and do some emotional and mental clearing to help release any trapped energy from this ridiculous procedure.

And thirdly, it's not your fault. Speak out and get help. And most of all love your ladies bits, however, they are, and reconnect with them lovingly.

You can't help the abuse that went on, but you can be on your body's side and learn to love your precious holes and labia or lack thereof, just as they are.

You are still a beautiful woman and powerful. Tune into the energetic precious holes, clitoris and flaps, they are still there. Whenever we lose a limb or any part of our physical body, the energy pattern remains intact. It won't grow again, but it will help to rebuild a truer connection to your body and may help mentally, to know that at some level, you are still intact.

\* \* \*

## Linguistic Interlude

We have covered the linguistic links to our bladder already, but here are a few more linked to our precious holes or where they lead to. Can you think of any more?

- *Fart-arsing about/Fannying about/Pussyfooting around/Beating around the bush.* Means not being direct or not getting straight to the point – **well I tell you now, I'm done with people beating about my bush!**

- *Douche/Douchebag.* Is an insult (the actual douche means showering up your vagina and douche-bag is where the fluid is held that gets sprayed up into the vagina. Do not use these, in my opinion, they are problematic).

- *Thunder-Thighs.* An insult to women with larger/fatter thighs.

- *Twat/Cunt/Pussy/Fanny/Minnie/Minge/Clunge.* These are all insults.

- *Dickhead/Prick/Dick/Cock/Bell-End.* These are all insults.

- *Arse/Arsehole/Butthead/Crackpot/Shit-for-brains.* These are all insults.

- *Bollocks/Crap/Shit/Bugger/Bum/Fuck.* Denote annoyance or anger.

- *Hysteria/Hysterical Women.* Derived from the word in Greek meaning uterus, and is used to denote madness or extreme emotional outbursts.

- *Slag/Slut/Prozie/Whore/Slapper/Hoe.* Words to insult women who have sex out of marriage or get paid for it, or who just have sex! If a man has multiple partners or sleeps around he is called a *Stud or a Gigolo. Er,* that's hardly offensive.

Ladies, it is perfectly normal and OK for you to have sex whenever, with whomever, and with as many partners as you like. Your body is yours to do with as you please, it just means you are human, although do be aware of the importance of safe sex.

## Chapter 5 Keynotes

- Other illnesses not related to the bladder directly can still be linked to a type of cystitis.

- Women's health issues are numerous and a nuisance but can usually be dealt with.

- Women's issues are not taboo, dirty, shameful, distasteful, or to be ignored. Speak about them and get the help you need.

- Let's no longer use our body parts as insults or to give offence. Let's restore respect and honour to the female anatomy in all areas including our language.

## Action! Interactive bit, it's your turn:

1. Do you have bladder issues, other than cystitis? If you are not sure, now is the time to call your doctor. I'm not kidding, do it now, and then write your appointment in your journal. You need to know what you are dealing with.

2. Write in your journal any feelings that came up reading this chapter.

3. If you have any of these bladder issues, or other women's health issues then consider what functional help you may be able to get, not just for the physical bladder but the energetic one too. Living with any of these traumatic issues may have caused energy blocks. It is a good idea to find help to release those.

4. Write in your journal any linguistic clues that you are aware of and the phrases you use regularly that incorporate body parts.

So, we are now even more aware of most conditions that can affect our bladders or precious holes.

We understand WHY the 25 types of cystitis happen.

We, therefore, understand how to start avoiding them too.

We are now wise.

So it's time to really understand HOW to avoid them in detail by getting to learn the all-important protocols that I devised for complete happy bladder health.

**This is the empowering part I mentioned in the title.**

Ready? Follow me as we are now leaving Part One.

We are going to slow it down a little as we review Part One, but then afterwards,

buckle up, Gorgeous, crank up the mixed-tape volume and let's zoom onto the juicy stuff!

**Yep, it's time for the A-Team!**

# Part One Highlights

As we take a well-earned pit-stop, let's mull over briefly what we discovered in the first part of our trip.

- I hope you are enjoying your free gifts.

- We established that this book is my opinion based on personal experience and research.

- We took an in-depth look at my experiences with the urological medical world & got you thinking about yours.

- We explored why bladders can become unhappy.

- We know what our waterworks and our precious holes look like inside and out. We even had a good gander in the mirror. Right?

- We have a basic understanding of metaphysics and how it may affect our bladder.

- We explored the linguistic links & are aware of our words.

- We discovered there are 25 types of cystitis.

- We have the wisdom of why cystitis happens.

- We have touched upon other issues that can affect the bladder and precious holes.

And now we are back in our car, driving through the tunnel as we arrive in Part Two.

# PART TWO

## The HOWS!
## Empowering solutions to avoiding all types of cystitis

You are taking the driver's seat.

## CHAPTER 6

# Building Your Bladder A-Team

Oh, this is the juicy bit. It's the potential life-changing part I mentioned before.

We now understand *exactly* what cystitis is, the 25 different possible types and how we can get them. We are appreciating our bladder and what makes it tick or tock.

In addition to already knowing how the 25 types come about and therefore how to avoid them, we are going to look at action steps to help keep all types of cystitis away.

So now, let's build your **A-Team**, bringing your A-Game daily to your bladder health. This is where we go into detail on how to treat your bladder right.

I have devised this information in what I call 'protocols'.

Protocols are action steps in certain areas in your life that can affect bladder health.

This is a fully functional guide to building continuous bladder health, turning your nemesis into your best friend. Love your bladder, recognise all it has gone through to work for you, probably un-thanked and possibly abused, even if you didn't realise it, and acknowledge that it is still trying to work well for you.

Cystitis is a signal that the bladder needs help.

It's time to be on your bladder's side.

You know most of the *whys*, so you are now *wise* on how we get cystitis of all different types, so now let's give you back control by delivering you the *hows*, specifically how to avoid them.

The good news is that most of the causes are avoidable. You are now in the driver's seat because remember, **knowledge is key**.

It is now your choice if you build a happy bladder team or a sad one.

Why not join me in life-after-cystitis, it rocks! Let's go.

# HOW TO AVOID CYSTITIS PROTOCOLS

### 1- Toilet Protocols

- **Loo roll**

Use white toilet paper as this sometimes means fewer dyes were used. Do not use a scented one, or one impregnated with oils or aloe vera. Plain, white cotton loo roll, keep it simple.

And what the hell was that loo paper that my school used? It was brown tracing paper! It smeared rather than mopped and ripped your skin apart. If your workplace or school still use this questionable loo roll, then bring your own. Maybe consider flinging the offensive item at the boss or headmaster. I'm kidding, kind of.

- **Using loo roll**

It is important to wipe from top to bottom. Wipe your urethra first, and then down over your vagina and round to the anus, not the other way around as we do not want to spread urine, faecal or period matter onto the urethra.

- **Toilet hygiene**

It's not enough to just wipe after a poo, not for the A-Team. To show you why try this experiment: after your next poo and usual wiping, pass your hand from the top to bottom, on all your holes, and right between the butt-cheeks, and then look at it.

It will have loo roll residue, sometimes obvious bits, but always minute pieces, even if you can't see them, you may feel them, like soft grit.

This dirty paper residue will, especially if you wear tight underwear or thongs, touch your urethra and vagina and with the friction of walking and sitting could be pushed up and into your bladder.

- **Post-poo cleaning**

Use a clean flannel, organic cotton preferred. Use clean water. I know this is obvious, but I want to be clear, if you are abroad and the tap water is not drinkable, then I wouldn't use it to wipe my precious holes.

Most of the time you will be at home or at work and trust the water, but if unsure, use bottled spring or mineral water. You can get it as cheaply as 17p for 2 litres in some shops in the UK or 99c for three litres in the USA or Europe.

**Tip:** bring a small bottle of water and clean flannel in a bag to work or whilst travelling, you can use a refillable bottle.

After wiping, use some of the bottled-water to rinse your bits over the toilet, then use one side of the flannel to soak and then wipe your bum with it, ensuring to spread your butt cheeks and really clean the anus, in one direction only, towards your back, not your other holes. Then, use the dry half of the clean flannel to dry your butt, no need to dry your urethra or vagina, we do not want to irritate. You can just pat it gently with the clean part of the flannel if really wet.

Get into a routine to have your shower after your poo. As you get healthier you should regulate and empty your bowels at similar times, so you can plan ahead.

I have mine usually within 10 minutes of waking up, so I wait until after my business and then have my shower.

Use a detachable showerhead, that preferably has a filter on to rinse your holes.

- **How to use the toilet**

Use a hygienic toilet that you are in charge of cleaning, like the one at home, ensuring to clean it with a loo-brush often. If you use products to flush with, that is OK, but ensure none is on the seat or splashing back up when you pee in it.

If it is a public toilet or one at work then wipe the seat with loo roll before sitting on it, and throw the paper into the bowl, to avoid splashbacks, you know what I mean, if you have a big poo sometimes as it hits the water, some will splash upwards and possibly onto your urethra and that is not a good idea.

If it is a dirty public toilet, oh hell, we've all been there, right? Then don't use it, take the risk of peeing outside somewhere. It's not ideal and I don't encourage it normally, but if you are a cystitis sufferer and you need a wee but the public toilet is full of germs, then put your bladder health first.

Ladies, for emergencies, do carry a 'She-Wee' with you which is a plastic, rubber or paper tube that you use as a penis, it's great fun and helps with not touching dirty toilet seats.

Men, you have a natural advantage of having your own penis, well done, Dude, what a genius design. When I was wheelchair-bound, I had one (**a 'She-Wee', not a penis!**), as it was easier than trying to find disabled toilets and not have to hold my pee too long. There is always a way and preparation is key.

Don't sit on the toilet after pooing for too long. Whilst on the loo our precious holes are relaxed and open. If you have cystitis and need to continue sitting on the loo, then wipe and flush and then sit back down.

I learnt the above from experience. I once got cystitis from sitting on the toilet too long and in the cold. I was at my grandparent's house and wanted to read my dragon book but my sister didn't want the light on, so I went to the loo and did my business, and continued sitting there for over an hour reading. By the end, I had a pee and it burned. I went downstairs and Mémé Lili heard me so she got up and made me a hot water bottle and a herbal tea. Bless her.

If you have diarrhoea it is especially important to clean properly as the germs from one precious hole can soon transmit to others.

It is a good idea to use loo roll to flush and open the public cubicle door too, because the people before wiped their butts, touched the chain, and then opened the door, before they got to wash their hands.

- **Actually weeing and pooing**

Give yourself time. Do not rush. Do not push your wee or poo out too hard or too fast. Take this quality time to do the job comfortably and properly.

It is important not to strain too hard as this could cause inflammation, or worse, a fallen bladder or piles. It is important also to ensure that you empty your bladder properly so that all the pee is out. Using a 'squatty potty' is great. I have one around my toilet. Use it each time you need a poo and also if you want to as you pee, as it helps us to be in a more natural position to evacuate our bowels and bladder.

Ensure to wash your hands with appropriate soap when possible and rinse properly, especially under fingernails and dry on a clean towel.

**Well done, you have had a successful A-Team toilet experience!**

I know, two pages to explain how to have a wee & poo! But the gold is in the details.

These protocols seem like a lot, but they don't take long and will become a part of your routine.

## 2- Daily Hygiene Protocols

I shower twice a day, or three times if I'm going out for the evening.

I shower in the morning after my toilet experience and once before going to bed.

I don't like overhead rain-showers, they don't have enough pressure to reach all of your body and you can't clean under your feet or up your butt. If you enjoy those, then make sure you rinse off using the handheld one that usually comes on the side. If there is none, you can use a plastic cup or small bucket to fill up from the shower to rinse with. You can also wet a clean flannel in the shower to have a proper rinse of your bits. Whilst I'm abroad I buy a large 5-litre mineral water bottle and leave it by the bathtub and after showering I use that to rinse off.

Now, best to remove the harsh chemicals from the water. Fit a shower-head that has a filter system. I have two special shower-heads, one on my shower and the other that I sometimes take travelling so that wherever I go, I have filtered water.

**Warning**: if a country is somewhere where water is not drinkable, I would still use it to shower with as these filters remove some small particles of lime-scale, of chlorine and fluoride, but they do not eliminate microbes, so in that instance, I would not put the shower anywhere near my holes, for that I would rinse with mineral water. And do not bathe in contaminated water or water that is not safe to drink remember if we can't digest it, our bladder walls can't touch it either.

After each poo, wash your hands and under your nails using a nailbrush. Nails are best kept short as under them is a great place for germs to set up home, there is little air circulation and the chances of touching or spooning up germs are plentiful.

Think of where your fingers touch during the day: rubbish, putting bins out, pet litter, your own poo and pee, sweat, germs in the air, food, chemicals in products, and of course, all outside surfaces, handrails, door handles, loo chains, public taps, money, light pulls, light switches, elevator buttons, telephone buttons, computer keyboards, cups, cutlery, glasses, clothes, pens, and other people. We all know about the 'free nuts in the bowl at the bar' issue, well, everything you touch, will have other people's germs on there too, perhaps traces of their poo, their pee, their sweat, their dead skin cells, their mucus. You get the picture.

Most of these are harmless because they are neutralised by our antibodies.

However, the fewer germs our antibodies have to combat, the stronger our immune system will be for responding to a nastier threat.

If you still have long nails, I do at times as I love them, then use a nail brush at least once at night before bed to ensure your fingers are truly clean.

And remember, your partner's hands have also touched all these things in the day, so he also needs to clean his hands with a nail brush and properly rinse off any soap before touching you down below. Simple.

## 3- Products Protocols

What you put on your skin will end up in your blood and bladder. It is important to choose wisely when kitting out your home. Check labels and look up some of the ingredients online.

It's shocking what goes into the everyday products that we use without a thought.

During my research I have come across: mascara with tarmac, yep what they put on the road; makeup with lead and mercury; eye creams with plastics, most creams have them; food dye with crushed-up insects; tampons with toxic chemicals; popular drinks and foods with nerve-gas, yes, what was used to kill people in gas chambers, and this in children's products too, more on that later; lipstick with whale blubber, yes they killed a whale so you can have red lips. This leads me to a huge subject on product selection: animal cruelty and slaughter for beauty.

A lot of products are not animal-friendly. When I was a vegan, I refused to spend any money supporting any trade that killed animals. This was when animal-friendly products were not popular and hard to find and cost four times the price.

I remember training for my motorbike license at university and spending way more for boots that were not made of leather but still tough enough for biking. I counted myself lucky I found them, but since then it is now so easy to find vegan clothing, food, and products.

When I did most of my research, the internet didn't exist. I didn't have a computer, I wrote my dissertations for my degree on paper, yep with a pen, the old fashioned way. This book is more rounded because of how I had to come by some of the information I'm now sharing.

The Internet is amazing and Google rocks, information is instant gratification, but searching through libraries, paper books, taking notes, interviewing people who had experience in what I was learning, and actually talking to brand manufacturers asking to see ingredients lists, has a connection that internet doesn't.

Anyway, I digress, back to products.

My anti-animal-abuse crusade made choosing safer products easier, back then few brands were totally animal-friendly. Some said they were 'our products are not tested on animals' but they still supported the industry by using raw materials from people who did test and abused animals.

I'm happy to say that since 2013 in the UK and EU if a cosmetic product states *animal-friendly* it must also cover the entire supply chain.

It may not be easy finding a brand that ticks all the boxes. So find one you love, that is animal-friendly and with the least chemicals as possible, or make your own, being mindful of the raw materials.

You can access my YouTube channel (https://www.youtube.com/channel/UCVHKRGdC7twLEVVIUMhkkxQ) for free demonstrations of how I make my own products or what I use.

Remember that everything and everyone involved in raw materials or end-products will have added their frequency to the mix. Animal and human abuse or slavery is never a good frequency for your health, especially not the bladder, given its energetic link to abuse and not feeling safe.

In the nutrition section, I will go into detail about why drinking milk is not good for your bladder at any level, as by then your knowledge of basic metaphysics will be well-grounded. You will see how the life and death of your food impact your energy.

You are what you eat and put on your skin, and also what that food ate and what those products are all made from.

It's deep, yes, and that is what I promised you. I would be doing you a disservice if I didn't rip open taboos and pour it all out for you to see for yourself.

If you still decide to use products or eat foods where animals were abused, please know that is OK too. This book isn't about veganism or animal welfare.

This book is about you and your bladder health. I want to ensure you have the facts then you decide, as it is about giving *you* back the power of your body and health.

Most household products include harsh chemicals, fake scents and general nasties. These are not human-friendly and yet we habitually touch them, wash in them, wear clothes that have been laundered and softened in them, sleep in bedsheets covered in them, brush our teeth with them, wash our floors, walls, surfaces, windows, you get the idea. Everything under your kitchen sink, bathroom, laundry room, or make-up box is relevant and needs investigation.

In the 'Products & Services Reference', linked as a free gift, I will tell you what brands I use and where to buy them from, so if you want the simple tried and tested way, then just copy me, or enjoy your own journey of discovery.

## 4- Sexual Protocols

This includes sex with a partner, several partners, masturbation and use of sex toys.

I repeat, because this is very important, *anything* that comes into contact with your urethra could end up in the bladder if not peed or washed out before it reaches its destination. Just as sperm strives for the womb lining, bacteria or candida strives for that bladder lining. You have been warned.

*Now suck it up (pun intended!) as this is a LONG but very important protocol.*

- **Pre-sex hygiene**
Drink a large glass of water to have a pee ready for after sex, this is important, do not be dehydrated.

We have to limit germ transference to build a strong A-Team.
Your partner also needs to follow the daily hygiene protocols before sex. If you don't know him, then be brave and have a shower before sex and encourage him to do the same. At the very least use a clean flannel and rinse your bits first.

**Top tip**: although not pleasant, and still problematic as going into the digestive tract from the top end, but employ **damage limitation**. Before I was brave enough to speak out or when I found it impossible to stick up for myself and say no when I wanted to, I sucked on his fingers and his penis hard before sex, (they didn't seem to mind), but it was my way of ensuring a clean-ish penis and less chance of infection transference in my bladder.

This is a real emergency tool, as a shower is best! But at a push, at least do that, it's **not A-Team, but at least employ damage limitation.**

Your own saliva carries your antibodies.

It is a good idea to have those on your partner before he penetrates you as your body will most likely take a little less offence to the intrusion if it has your saliva on it.

Of course, at this point, ensure your saliva is clean by brushing your teeth with appropriate toothpaste, and rinsing and gargling well. Do not use your saliva if you have a cold sore, a mouth/throat infection or have been kissing someone that does.

Knowing you are both hygienic may help you enjoy sex more, let go of inhibitions and most partners then say that was the best sex ever. So, see sexual protocol as foreplay. Entice him in the shower but don't let him penetrate you as we don't want soap or water going up there, make sure he is clean, then move it to the bedroom.

If you have a regular partner, then do have the talk, tell them how you no longer wish to suffer from any type of cystitis and explain how you can get it and how important sexual protocol is to you. Tell him or her that if you feel more relaxed during sex because you know you are both clean, then you both will have a better time. Look up *tantric sex*, if you want a deeper connection. Make sexual hygiene protocol a ritual.

Ask your regular partner to read this book, or at the very least the sexual protocol section. If they can't make the time or the effort to know what you need for your sexual health, then they have no business touching you.

Obviously, this won't happen on a one-night stand! In those cases, it is up to you to apply as much damage limitation as possible.

**Command respect: you are worth it.**

- **Pubic Hair**

The A-Team waxes when needed, so every 8 weeks or before. You are in charge of your pubes and you decide, not your partner, not society, and not any taboos associated with personal hygiene.

When I first started waxing (trust me, go to a professional with plenty of experience!), I had comments like, 'oh, only porn stars get Hollywoods. What do you want to do that for? It's natural to have body hair'.

Now it doesn't bother me because it's no one else's business how I treat my body, except for yours right now, because I promised to be transparent and vulnerable on our road-trip to help impart crucial knowledge.

It is up to your partner about how they treat their body, but you can suggest that it would be better for you if they did wax or at least shave regularly, so that you are not invaded by a deep black forest of potential nasties each time you have sex and less chance of choking on that rogue pube that has manifested in your mouth or twisted itself around your tonsils.

If your partner is not prepared to man up on his sexual hygiene, then put your bladder health first and refuse to have sex with him, he will soon change his mind, or you will split up sooner and do yourself a favour.

Stand your ground, anyone willing to touch you should respect you.

Simple. It has taken me decades to understand that, but now that I have, it's a different ball game.

So, we have discussed how to prepare for sex, hygiene, and being open about your desire for cleanliness and short, or non-existent pubes, and good oral hygiene.

Now let's move on to actual sex, the intercourse sub-protocol.

- **Intercourse**

A-Team has to involve being fully present. I used to do several things that are told-tell signs that I was not in the moment during sex or that I was with the wrong guy:

1- Think of a shopping list for next week's meals.

2- Think of my to-do list for the next day.

3- Fake noises and enjoyment so that it would be over quicker.

4- Recoil inside to his touch and wish I was somewhere else.

OK, so I needed a lot of work to get where I am today and I'm hoping this book will help speed up that learning curve for you if you have similar issues.

For sexual health and heightened enjoyment, it is important to have that body connection, to listen to the signs. Your body knows all the answers, even to questions you don't know to ask.

Being present means breathing deeply, allowing oxygen into your cells to help relax muscles and feed the brain that is building up high levels of dopamine and endorphins (happy chemical, ecstasy and relaxants). Being present will help your system deal with the influx and make it more pleasurable.

It will also mean that you are connecting on a deeper level with your partner, making sex more of a treat rather than a chore.

Yes, I know, I really had issues and questionable partners!

The bladder can relax when you are present. It knows you have its back, you are in control and not off with the fairies or in the virtual shops whilst being intruded.

Yes, sex is natural, but for a female, or a man receiving anal sex, the body is being invaded. It is intruded by things that, in the anus at least, have no business being there. I'm not judging, just explaining that our reproductive systems are designed to have a penis inside the vagina to procreate, that's it.

No other hole was designed to take penis or fingers, and so to the body, it is an attack, even if you are enjoying it.

So your full presence will send reassurance signals and it will relax more, helping to reduce injury or over-sensitivity.

Be aware that your bladder is being bashed and it doesn't like that.

Something as simple as before sex, sending a message to the bladder saying:

'hey, bladder buddy, you are about to get battered a bit, but no worries, nothing will be coming up the urethra, all is clean and the rest of the body will enjoy it and soon endorphins are coming your way which you like, who doesn't? So hang in there, all is well, I got your back.'

Yes, I know, it's bonkers talking to your body parts, but why not?

I think you know me by now: I'm not all that conventional.

**Note:** If you have IC or menopausal issues, then it may help to use a natural lubricant before sex and I recommend organic raw coconut oil. Do not push *anything* into the urethra, this is for the flaps and vagina only, and if needed.

- **Anal Sex**

Use skin-friendly lubrication to avoid skin breaking or too much irritation resulting in inflammation. The best may not a commercial one as it may contain chemicals, but if you do, go for an organic water-based one, but perhaps try a natural one such as a high-quality aloe vera gelly may work well or raw organic coconut oil.

Do not use soap, yoghurt, scented lubricants, honey or chocolate spread…

Do not go from one hole to the other (anus to vagina or mouth). Leave the butt until last or use a condom for anal sex, then remove it before continuing with vaginal sex, or moving onto another partner, or use a fresh condom.

Remember fingers count too, so if a cheeky-pinkie goes in your bum, don't allow that into your vagina, or suck that finger after so that at least you have cleaned off any faecal matter or candida before it touching your precious holes. Yes, it is in your mouth then, but your mouth has antibodies, your stomach has strong acid and alkaline juices, and there is way more chance your body neutralising germs or candida via the whole digestive tract, but your urethra and bladder have no such defences, as they are designed as an *exit* only.

If you don't enjoy anal sex, find the courage to have that conversation with your partner and avoid it altogether.

If you suffer from IBS, colitis, have an inner-bag, leaky gut or other intestine issues, do not have anal sex, you will be going totally against your body and abusing it.

If you do enjoy anal sex, either as a man or a woman, then take precautions to limit any transference.

Adhering to these protocols will help to lessen the risk of cross-contamination.

- **After sex**

Go to the toilet straight after sex, don't snuggle yet.

Gently allow the pee to come, even if it's just a drop or two. Don't push too hard as all your precious holes and tubes will be inflamed to some level. Then wash, if not a shower then with a clean flannel. Rinse, water is usually enough, I don't like using any soap on the vulva area and wipe, as always, from front to bottom.

Please avoid those fem-washes, or wet-wipes as they are not cystitis or skin-friendly.

I use an aloe vera liquid soap in the shower, that's it, but water is enough on the urethra or vagina, but soap is necessary on the butt.

Drink a large glass or more of room-temperature spring or mineral water.

Remember that sex will irritate the urethra and vagina due to the trauma, the physical act of bashing, and you may have a mild cystitis feeling, but if all was clean, then this will usually settle down, especially if you drink water and have a gentle wee after sex.

If you are with a new partner having lots of sex then this could also increase the risk of cystitis as the body doesn't have time to recuperate. This is *honeymoon cystitis.*

Do not leave it too long before peeing, even if you feel you don't need to go as even just a few drops will help flush out any foreign bodies, tiny pieces of loo paper, dead skin cells, pubes, semen or germs before making their way into the bladder.

Water will hydrate it and keep it moist and filling up with fresh pee ready to push out again by the morning, to ensure no rogue intruders are making their way near the sphincter from the outside.

Hydration is also an anti-inflammatory and will help you recover from sex quicker.

Place your hands on your bladder, thank it and love it. Then relax, stop thinking and go and have that snuggle and good night sleep. All is well.

Don't allow your partner to touch you again down below until he/she has washed too.

- **Sexual energy lingers**

It is worth mentioning that energy plays a huge role in post-sex. For a man, it is natural (not moral or kind, but a design flaw) to want to spread his seed. He enters the female and once he has left and washed, that's it, her energy is off him, he moves on, or stays with her but is not 'polluted' by her energy.

For a woman, however, it is very different. By design, we select the one male that we fall in love with or at least have strong feelings towards as our hormones choose him to reproduce with. Somewhere deep within us, our cells think that man is the one and only, who will look after us, feed us, protect us and help us bring up children.

Even if sex is just for pleasure or a one-night stand, it is natural for women to be more emotionally attached than the man.

A male's energy remains within the woman's field for about 1 year, or way longer if we don't clear the mental issues linked with splitting up or the horror of being raped.

A woman is intruded, she is possessed by the male energy field deep to her core, to her creativity hub (vagina and womb) and if he releases his sperm inside there too, that stuff lingers for days physically, and a lot longer metaphysically.

So even if you have a one night stand, that male energy will be with you for a while.

It is worth remembering that before deciding who to have sex with.

*Phew, right that's the sexual protocol done. I'm glad we had the talk. Moving on...*

## 5- Food Hygiene Protocol

Repetition is key. You can chant it with me by now: everything you eat, drink, inhale or touch will at some point come in contact with your bladder walls or your colon. So, if you eat contaminated food, that germ will be having a field day in your system, irritating your insides leaving infection behind, especially on your bladder walls.

If you think food or drink is dodgy, then don't have it, never mind about being too embarrassed or too shy to say anything and end up eating stuff to be polite. That will not help you when you are doubled-up in pain with diarrhoea and bladder cramps.

Remember that being *too nice* is not good for you, especially your bladder.
Stand up for your health.

The primary role of food is fuel.
We eat to help our body function. We eat enough non-foods as it is (gluten, corn, dairy, sugars, chemicals, over-manufactured, junk, trans-

fats…) that destroy our systems on a regular basis, so let's avoid infected-food as much as possible.

**Food hygiene is**: ensuring your kitchen surfaces are clean; your hands are clean; your cutlery and serving dishes are clean; your fridge is clean and has designated shelves for raw meat and other foods; when you touch raw meat you wash your hands and change utensils before preparing other foods; you use a different chopping board for raw meat and veggies; if you rinse raw chicken or meat under the sink, ensuring no splash-backs go onto your crockery sitting on the drying section; when you clean kitchen surfaces, that you don't do it when food or drinks are out, especially if using spray cleaners that are air-born then land on your food, be mindful not to contaminate the food or water in your pet bowls either.

Look out for food hygiene certifications in restaurants and be the person who complains if there is hair in your soup or if meals look or smell wrong, don't be embarrassed, you are the paying client and they have to provide safe food.

I once got food poisoning within 20 minutes of eating my chicken meal whilst out at university with my friends. I was embarrassed and got a taxi back to the flat with the excuse that I was tired. I missed the night out and I didn't complain or tell anyone, because I felt dirty. I got cystitis too because of it. Don't do that. If you get ill at a restaurant, tell the management and make a big deal about it. I would now.

And worth mentioning again, food is fuel, it is not part of sex. Food as a pre-sex enjoyment ritual, such as a romantic meal, a glass of champagne, or feeding each other sensually is great, but do avoid rubbing it on your bits.

Food should only go one way into our digestive tract, through the mouth, where your saliva can start the digestive process, then stomach, organs, intestines, colon or kidneys, bladder and then out.

**Urethras, vaginas, and anuses should all have no entry signs.**

And, I will mention again here, that anything that goes into your mouth potentially affects your bladder, so that means *anything*, not just food and drink, but body parts too. At this stage, consider breaking the habit of biting your nails. Remember what lives under your nails. Luckily, we have amazing antibodies in our mouth, so most are neutralised before hitting the bladder walls, but not all, and not all the time. It's still a risk factor in bladder and throat health.

The A-Team doesn't bite nails.

## 6- Clothing Protocol

What your clothes are made of is important. Most are man-made materials created in a lab with all sorts of nasties potentially including petrol, plastics, glues, chemicals, toxic dyes, and pesticides.

They also contain energy frequencies of the people and animals, whether working animals or tested subjects, involved in making it.

Energies from all involved, from harvesting the raw materials to the factory to the shop assistant that sells it to you. So, do consider the social, humane, and animal welfare issues of your clothing, because if a person or an animal was enslaved or hurt during any of the processes then you are associating with abusive leftover frequency.

Remember that those energies tend to make a home in bladders, especially if your waterworks is your weak area.

Once awakened to basic metaphysics, we can no longer hide or believe that we are not all connected, that energy doesn't matter, and that at some level we are not affected by what we eat, use, or wear. Allowing abuse in any way into our lives is inviting it into our energy field and our bodies.

Even if we don't personally abuse that animal, rip apart a wild habitat, destroy the Amazon forest, create child labour, or subject animals to a life of misery in labs or cages, if we use our money to buy such a product lining the pockets of those who do, then we are a huge part of the abuse equation: there is no getting away from that.

**We vote with our money.**
Choose wisely how you spend yours. You deserve the best.

By treating yourself right, you also treat the planet right. The more of us who are doing that, then the more these abusive industries will be forced to change because right now, they only think of profit and power.

Take your power back, give your money to companies who respect nature, and you.

We can change the world, one person at a time, one decision at a time, and one purchase at a time.

I know, it's not easy to find out what you are buying exactly, but it is getting easier as more of us demand it. If there is a choice of buying organic, do so.

If a product specifies 'animal-friendly', choose that brand.
Make your own products and clothing if you can.

Remember, it's not about changing everything at once.
Start with buying organic cotton underwear, towels and bed linen.

It is not easy to think of everything, that is my job here as the author. Your job is to read, let this information sink in and make different choices as you go along.

Small changes are effective, it's the compound effect.

I'm not saying chuck out all your clothes and start again, I'm saying from now on be mindful of what you buy. I'm not saying you have to research each brand before making a decision, but awareness will help you choose the best items, and you will attract better clothes if that is your wish.

It is about damage limitation, so for some clothing make a change now, and I would say the most important is what touches your precious holes. So with underwear, chuck out polyester, satin, frilly, tight knickers and definitely any thongs or strings.

I don't care how sexy they look, they do contribute to vaginal thrush, itchy anus, and of course, cystitis.

Right, so ditch the strings, in any case, it is generally known that men think a woman with no knickers as more of a turn on.

And tough shit if your partner wants to see you in thongs, let him get cystitis and itchy bits and then see how attached he is to sexy knickers: your health comes first.

## Linguistic Interlude

I know I just used *tough shit* as an expression, using body waste in my language but it came out naturally so I left it, to show more awareness of expressions we use without thinking.

*There are a few others in the book, can you spot them?*

**Note:** if you are going to wear trousers or jeans, then do wear big knickers made of organic cotton if possible, as trouser material will come into contact with your bits, but limit the use of a tight anything around there.

Adopt wearing flowy skirts or loose cotton trousers. In summer, if wearing a long skirt, what is the point in underwear? Go 'commando', allowing the air to free flow and with no chaffing at all.

Give your bits a holiday too as we are not designed to have that area closed off. So going commando gives your precious holes and delicate flaps time to be free.

Wearing underwear when not necessary is like chaining yourself to your office desk. Especially, if you are someone who wears pyjamas too, then your precious holes never get fresh air. Sleep naked on organic cotton sheets: that is the A-Game.

Organic cotton or bamboo is best for your underwear, and if not organic, then at least high-quality cotton, what I call 'big girls' pants, with plenty of material and quite loose around the gusset, with room for air to circulate and to avoid too much chafing.

The same thing for leggings, source cotton not polyester, most will have elastane that's normal but choose cotton or hemp as the main material.

Where possible, choose organic and natural dyes.

Natural materials are cotton, linen, hemp, bamboo, wool, silk, and leather (but animal skin comes with abuse energy). Bear in mind that the fabric industry is taxing on the environment, and it takes a lot of water to cultivate cotton, so even among the natural materials, environmental issues are still worth considering.

The happier your clothes' energy, the less impact they had on others and the planet, the less abusive the energy will be linked to them, so if you can, choose wisely.

The most economical and less planet-damaging is organic hemp and organic bamboo because these grow fast and are easily replanted.

It will be difficult to bring your full A-Game in this section but do make some changes to your wardrobe. Also, notice how you feel wearing happier clothes.

Start appreciating what you put on your skin, and what you dress your body with, because it all counts.

## 7- Nutritional Protocol

Do not rely on doctors for nutritional advice or diets. They have very little to no training in nutrition, and what they have learnt has been (in my opinion) erroneous as they consider dairy and grains to be a normal part of human requirements.

When my Dad was diagnosed with lung cancer, I asked the doctor if he thought nutritionally we could do something to help him. I knew there was, of course, but my Dad was very much respectful of authority and of the generation that if a doctor says something then it must be so. I'm not of that generation, thank F.

His doctor laughed and said "No, he can eat and drink whatever he wants because food doesn't make any difference to his health. The chemotherapy is what will help."

I shut up as there was no point in arguing with such a Beep, but my heart sank as I knew my Dad would take that on board. The chemotherapy, radiotherapy and all the other hideous drugs did not help him or save him. I'm not saying proper nutrition would have either, it was his time to go, but it may have helped prolong his life or support his body in the fight.

The point I'm making is don't rely on medics for knowing what to eat and drink.

Would you trust a mechanic with your precious car if he had no clue about what to fuel it with if he had no real training on oil, water, petrol or their effects on the car? No? Shocker. Then don't trust a doctor with your body or rather nutrition either.

I found that **food-combining** helped me with digestive issues and get rid of candida overgrowth. I didn't mix proteins and carbohydrates in the same meal. We have different digestive enzymes to digest proteins and sugars and I found if I mixed those in the same meal, my digestion was slower and food fermented more in my gut as a result. When you are not on a strict anti-candida diet and you are having carbs and sugars do not mix them with proteins. For example, for lunch, I had jacket potato with beans and salad (all carbs/sugar and neutral) and for dinner I had chicken and stir fry green veggies and onions (protein and neutral).

**Inflammation/swollen tissue causes bladder pain as well as most diseases ending with -*itis* and therefore limiting foods and drinks that cause inflammation is a great idea.**

The A-Team avoids all inflammatory foods, especially those linked to food sensitivity or cystitis. Please note though that in this modern age it will be ridiculously difficult to avoid these forever, so it is OK to have times when we indulge. I know I do.

When I'm strict on my zero-sugar or sweetener campaign I'm really good, and this enables me to increase my fulcrum for the times when I apply the 'Ah, fuck it mode it's (enter excuse here) and eat and drink what I fancy. More on *fulcrums* later.

**A-Team says no to inflammatory/acid-forming foods:**

- Gluten
- Wheat
- Corn
- Palm Oil
- Soya
- Dairy
- Eggs
- Sugars (remember there are over 50 names for sugar)
- Too much fruit
- Processed Meats/Fish/Junk Food
- Too much meat even the good stuff
- Caffeine
- Chocolate
- Cranberry
- Tomatoes, chilli, peppers, potato, aubergine
- Fizzy drinks/Squash/Cordial
- Sweeteners
- Alcohol
- Cigarettes/tobacco
- Pesticides/fungicides/chemicals
- Aluminium foil or aluminium food containers
- Clingfilm and plastic food containers
- Microwaves
- And limit your fruit intake

Say yes to anti-inflammatory foods, also known as alkalising. They feed your gut bacteria (microbiome). No need to take pre or probiotics if you just eat the right foods and your body will create its own, however in a society where the soil is depleted and we do also indulge in 'negative food', it would be wise to take good quality supplements and probiotics.

Always choose organic or home-grown fruit, vegetables, herbs, spices, and grains.

For fish, choose wild-caught, not farmed. If it is not stated that it was wild-caught, then it wasn't.

For meat, not just organic, but an animal fed a healthy diet they were designed to eat, for instance, cows eat organic grass, that's it, not cereal or meat pellets.

Hens are designed to peck around eating insects, plants, flowers, not factory-made pellets or to live cramped in a cage.

Fish are designed to eat wild seaweed, coral, and smaller fish, not chicken or grain pellets, and swim freely in rivers or oceans, not cramped in farms.

Humans are designed to eat wild meat, wild fish, organic seeds, nuts, organic vegetables and some fruit, and plenty of clean water. We are not meant to consume manufactured or chemical-laden stuff that is technically not food.

**Let's explain more why your gut microbiome is so important.**

We have two opposite beasts living in our gut. They are conscious intelligent collectives. One based on yeasts, mainly called Candida (yeasts and bad bacteria) and the other is a colony of various 'Good Gut Flora' such as Lactobacillus acidophilus and Bifidobacterium bifidumare.

Lactobacillus acidophilus is crucial and it also helps fight candida not only in the gut but also in the vagina, cervix, and urethra, as it produces lactic and acetic acids that stop the growth of certain bacteria and yeasts.

*You* are the colony that you feed the most.

This isn't symbolic: it is literal.

'Candida' is alive and has a strong controlling voice that talks directly to your brain. You may call this a *sugar monster* or that voice that forces you to eat more sugar-based foods. It is a bully if it becomes out of control or overfed.

'Good Gut Flora' is the quieter voice that asks for healthy food and lifestyle. These guys are the most important and we need way more of these than the yeast colonies.

Which beast will you feed most?

**If you feed mostly the candida colony this may encourage:**

- Inflammatory diseases (-itis)
- Foggy brain
- Bad breath
- Weight gain
- Depression
- Anxiety
- Illnesses
- Bad thoughts and choices
- Anger, mood swings
- Sugar crashes and cravings
- Cancer
- Over-acidic conditions

The candida preferred diet is acid-forming:

- Sugars
- Gluten
- Grains
- Additives
- Chemicals
- Microwaved food
- Junk food
- Alcohol
- Cigarettes
- Dairy
- Stress
- Drama
- Gossip
- Negativity
- Dampness
- Negative, heavy emotions and dark thoughts
- Dirty sex

**If you feed mainly the Good Flora colony (the pretty flowers!)**

This will most likely be your experience:

- Happiness
- Clarity
- Good health
- Good energy
- Vibrancy
- Fluidity and flexibility
- Good thoughts and good choices
- Healthy weight

- Love
- Hope, drive, passion

Their preferred diet is:

- Alkaline forming foods
- All organic
- Vegetables
- Green smoothies and juices
- Organically grown aloe vera gel drink
- Organic nuts (not peanuts or cashews)
- Natural water and plenty of it
- Meditation
- Deep breathing/plenty of oxygen
- Positive thoughts and smiling
- Movement in nature/gentle exercise
- Healthy fats (olives, nuts, avocado, seeds).
- Lemon
- Anti-inflammatory foods
- Mindful eating

A useful supplement to take would be *Saccharomyces Boulardii*. It is yeast that does not colonize our system but fights others that do for the sugar. In other words, it grabs candida and gets it out of your system as it passes.

We are overfed and yet malnourished. Most of what we eat is not classed as food but toxins. Our bodies are forced to operate on not enough nutrients that it should be getting from good true sources of food.

## Comedy Interlude:

Here is a great example of how my microbiome speaks to me. I'm letting you see a sneak peek into my inner dialogue. You know I talk to everything by now and yes I'm totally nuts. Awesome.

Picture the scene, I'm shopping in the supermarket my trolley full of good yummy stuff such as green veggies for smoothies, salads, lemons, nuts, seeds and wild-caught salmon. I'm feeling rather good.

Then I spot the chocolate and biscuit aisle.

I quickly walk past it, ignoring it, but it's too late, my yeast colony has also spotted it. They have now lassoed my brain and taken over.

Yeast (aka Yeast Beast – YB): uh, what do you think you doing?

Me: Uhm, nothing, tra-la-la, just walking about.

YB: liar. You're shopping and you missed the sugar goodies. Go back and turn into that aisle, you loser.

Me: no thanks. I have all that was on my list, I'm good to go.

*Making my way to the checkout. Damn, I'm stuck behind an old lady who just stopped dead in the middle of the aisle.*

YB: well, you can't wait here forever, go back and down the sugar aisle, it is the quickest route to the exit.

Me: damn it. OK, but I'm not buying anything.

YB. *smirks*. That's OK, we can just look as you stroll by.

Good Bacteria (aka GB): that's not a good idea, Mummy. You know what happened the last times.

YB: shut up, Dumb-arse, go back to sleep.

Me: *sigh.*

*We walk down the aisle. As soon as I do, as if by magic, I'm bombarded by images of all the sugary treats that I have loved in my time, memories of my grandma giving me chocolate spread on waffles, my other nan, ginger biscuits.*

Me: oh, come on! YB, this isn't fair, you said we would just look, not bombard my inner sight with images of such happy times.

YB: *clearly rummaging in the memory banks.* Don't know what you mean.

Me: damn it! They have an offer on orange Kit-Kats. *I stop the trolley.*

GB: Oh, for the love of firm faeces, don't stop!

YB *pushes the good bacteria, sits on his face and puts on his charming syrupy voice*: ooo look, a bargain. Come on, you know you love a bargain.

*I put one in the trolley and walk away.*

*YB lassoes my neck and yanks me back, chucks out the one chocolate bar and puts in the multiple pack of 6.*

YB: well, you see I'm just looking after your finances. If you look at the price per bar from a bulk packet, you are saving so much. Don't be ripped off buying just one.

Me: well, you have a point there.

*GB slaps his own face and puts his hands over his eyes, like the cute monkey emoji.*

YB: well, now look at that big bag of Minstrels, you love those, remember the time when… (He inserts times when I enjoyed that treat).

Me: oh, yes I do. I'd forgotten about that.

*I grab a bag and put it in.*

*Right, now we must really get to the checkout.*

GB: about time, yes, Mummy, run; save yourself!

YB: don't be such a drama queen, GB: it's only a bit of sugar.

GB: and sweeteners, gluten, chemicals, fat, shit. Not to mention one bite will lead to a full out sugar orgy.

*I try to not let that image take hold which is hard after the film 'Sausage Party'.*

Me: you both have good points. So let's compromise. We got lots of goodies for you, GB and we got plenty for you too, YB.

*A murmur of agreement.*

YB: Uhm, look the checkout queues are so long! Let's just hang around, you know how you hate standing in line. Why not look up this aisle?

GB: oh, how convenient it's the cereals aisle. Don't do it, Mummy, look at the toilet roll and general cleaning aisle next to it instead...

Me: well, the cereals is the closest aisle, to be fair...

GB *slaps his face again.* There is nothing fair about this ambush. I knew you'd be on his side.

Me: I'm not taking sides, I'm just innocently going up the nearest aisle.

*Images of when I loved these cereals bombard me. I can smell the chocolate Ready Brek that my nan used to make. I can feel the crunch of the Crunchy*

*Nut Cornflakes and remember the advert on TV that made me laugh. I'm smiling at all these memories, mesmerised in my own inner world.*

*YB doesn't say anything but gets his big "Fuck it" card and uses it to shovel stuff in the trolley as I walk by. By the time I get to the checkout, I can barely see the green veggies, squished under the pot of chocolate spread, waffles and variety of cereals.*

*GB has given up and almost lost the will to live.*

*YB is so out of control I can barely call him back to us. I see him as a rampaging beast, a naughty little critter pulling shit off the shelves and throwing it in the trolley, whilst letting out evil screams and making rude signs at other shoppers.*

*We get to the checkout. Mountains of so-called food beep past the till. When did the deep pan cheese-filled crust pizza get in there? Chips? I don't even like chips. Finally we get to the squished lettuce bags, the celery and other good stuff.*

*I nervous-giggle and explain to the check-out lady that kids are coming over.*

*Got to have the sweeties! Oh, but look so much healthy stuff for me.*

*She smiles.*

*I wonder if she can tell I'm lying and don't have kids?*

*I shuffle my way to the car and shove it all in quickly, hiding my sins.*

*Then YB chimes in.*

YB: Uhm, why not put the Minstrels in your handbag, don't want to squish them in all that celery.

*Whilst driving home, the Minstrels are literally calling my name.*

Minstrels: Jennnifer, Jeeeeeeeennnnnnnifer, I'm here... you know you want me.

*I can't concentrate, the thought of eating them is all-encompassing.*

*YB quietly reminds me that I'm such a good driver, and it's not good to be distracted whilst on the road. I should really eat the Minstrels. Afterall, it is their raison-d'être and I will be doing them a disservice not enjoying them.*

*As I reach mid-point in my journey, the chocolate bastards have gone. I lick my lips.*

YB: I said you would be pleased if you listened to me. But oh, wait! Now you don't have Minstrels anymore for your TV night. *He looks genuinely concerned.*

Me: well, I still got the other stuff in the boot.

YB: Forget that trash in the trunk. I think we need gas. Look, stop there is a gas station. *Evidently, YB is part American which is another reason he gets to me, as I love the accent.*

Me: I still have well over ¾ of a tank left.

YB: yes, but you never know, what if (he inserts dangerous scenarios where I could run out of gas.) And you are such a good driver. Good drivers think ahead.

Me: best be safe then.

*I stop off and fill up with petrol and stand in line to pay.*

YB: Well, that's embarrassing, it's less than £4 worth of gas. Why not spend a little more? It's hardly worth queuing up for such a small amount. Oh: they do Minstrels.

Me: OK.

*By this point, I've lost any kind of authority. I pick up the Minstrels.*

*At the till I'm reminded by YB's oozy voice that the Cadburys Cream Eggs are out.*

YB: they only come out once a year. You know how much you love those.

*He starts to show me all the images of when I had cream eggs.*

Me: Oh, for fuck's sake! OK.

*I smile awkwardly as I snapped out loud, forgetting that other people can't see or hear the Yeast Beast.*

*By the time I get home, the cream eggs have gone, merging in my tummy along with the dead Minstrels.*

*But I still have the new bag of Minstrels for my TV night: result.*

GB: Well, there goes my food.

Me: what do you mean, look at this lovely greenery here in the fridge, it looks amazing. I will have a nice healthy green smoothie before I have the YB food.

GB: uh, we'll see. You will ignore my food until it goes rancid in the fridge and you are forced to throw it out, and get angry at yourself for wasting good food again.

Me: *harrumph*. Oh, don't be like that. It will be different this time.

*By the time I go to bed, I feel bad and GB was right and the green and healthy stuff is still sitting in the fridge, sell-by-date rapidly going off.*

*And I feel sick after the pizza, waffles with chocolate spread and the Minstrels, and I'm not sure how many orange Kit-Kats remain in the bargain pack.*

*YB has finally shut up. I can hear him snoring, rolling around with a huge stomach, farting and being a general pest.*

*I can see GB getting smaller as he dies under YB's expanding foul mass.*

Me: I feel really sick and fat. I promise tomorrow will be different. Tomorrow, I will be really good.

*GB sighs and rolls his eyes. He knows that ain't gonna happen. When the candida has me crumpled up in pain again, I will then go on an anti-candida campaign and reset, being totally on GB's side, but until then… YB has won another battle.*

*I try and turn my bloated belly over to sleep.*

Me: one day, you yeast bastards, I will win the war.

* * *

I hope you enjoyed that microbiome interlude! It reinforces that we can at times feel overpowered by the yeast. Candida is real, it has a voice and it does talk directly to our brain. Being aware of that will help give you control back.

Don't give up.

As I said, it's OK to have those days, just keep going and make some changes. At least ensure to feed the good bacteria too. So even if you have a lot of crappy food, also have some aloe vera and green smoothies too, and maybe end the night with a glass of water and bicarbonate of soda or lemon to help alkalise your system.

Organic food in toxic plastic, in aluminium cans, and heated in a microwave almost defeats the objective. **The A-Team** is about wild meat and fish, and fruit and vegetables that are grown naturally having sourced the seeds correctly and no packaging. I realise that in this current world this is unlikely for most people, it used to be a few generations back, but lately the world has gone mad.

Be the person who makes that change. Live in this world with a foot in the new world we wish to create, one with reasonably-priced natural healthy foods and no abuse.

So, the A-Team is not totally realistic in the nutrition field, but do make some changes and deploy some damage limitation tactics.

Unfortunately, governments and the food industry are mainly about profit – money, money, money. So, adding sugars in food helped keep us under their control because sugar is addictive so we want more.

That is why sugar has been introduced in foods, even in foods it has no business being in. It is even in the wild-caught smoked salmon I used to buy, I contacted them about it and they said it was necessary to keep it fresh. This is rubbish, as before we used sugar, food was still fresh, and salt brine is sufficient in most cases, and so I sourced a smoked salmon brand that didn't use sugar: **we vote with our money.**

You will notice that organic foods can be more expensive than regular and that is largely because it is cheaper to make fake foods than real foods. It is also because some governments subsidise some food industries to encourage the masses to buy certain brands. **The A-Team** does not get bullied in this way.

In the UK, we now have a *sugar tax* but only on soda/fizzy drinks, so the government is penalising companies (who pass the debt onto us) for adding extra sugar to their drinks and so the government is still profiting, as now if we choose sugar, we pay extra, but naturally sugar-free foods are still more expensive.

Getting a sugar-tax was awesome for awareness of how bad sugar is for us, but they should not allow the companies to pass it to the consumer. And there needs to be a sugar tax on *all* food and drink. Still, it is a great step in the best direction.

The government needs to give the money that the sugar tax creates to organic food producers, hence subsidising health, that would be the thing to do and the more of us refusing to eat sugar and unreal foods, the more they will listen.

I was angry at a well-known brand of pasta tomato sauce in a jar. It was the same brand, the same size, with the same ingredients, except in one the sugar had not been added. The 'no added sugar' jar was *twice* the price. They were penalising me for making a healthier choice because they know they make more money if sugar is in the food due to its addictive nature. I didn't want the one with sugar but I refused to pay double for having no sugar.

So I took a picture of them and put it in my healthy food tribe on Facebook, and of course, I won't buy that brand again. I purchased organic tomatoes, onions and herbs, and made my own sauce, which was the healthiest and cheapest option anyway. I'm hoping now that the sugar-tax is in place, it will evolve so that the 'no added sugar' products will be cheaper, and the sugar ones more expensive or banned.

If we keep paying for cheap food, then we will keep getting cheap food, and that pushes the price of real food way up, to the point only people who really care about their health and animal welfare will pay.

We can stop that. Every time you put your health first, it helps to set a trend and send a crucial message. With the help of social media now, companies are more aware and it does give the consumer a much louder voice, especially if you are an influencer or have a huge following.

So if you stop buying a product due to its sugar or chemical content, do tell the company why you are no longer a customer and share that brand on Facebook, warning others of its unhealthiness and promote those that are healthier.

As I said, we can take our power back.

**Example**: chicken, a popular choice of meat. You can buy a large chicken for £4 in a supermarket or you can buy a real chicken (organic, free-range and fed a natural diet, been cared for, had a happy life and then killed as humanely as possible) and pay up to £15. The difference is ridiculous. The reason why cheap chicken is cheap is that they have totally abused the hen, it has been fed antibiotics and chemical-laden pellets and not been allowed out to use its muscles at all, and has been treated abysmally then slaughtered before its time in a horrific manner.

Oh, my! Now, that you understand basic metaphysics and that energy begets similar energy, what frequency do you think you are attracting if your own flesh and blood are laden with animal abuse, chemical warfare and if your money is being used to encourage this behaviour?

Quite simply put, the cheap chicken is fake, not actual food. The organic free-range chicken is real food.

**No matter how cheap that non-food is, it still costs too much.**

You are not comparing like for like. We may as well say that buying a plastic chicken that kids play with in their pretend kitchen is cheaper than buying a real chicken and eat that.

Eating the real chicken has cost you more money, but has increased your health by providing bio-available protein and other goodness, potentially increasing your lifespan and cleared up your aura frequency.

It also sends a message to the food industry that animal abuse is no longer tolerated.

Eating cheap meat has cost you less money but has cost you way more: it has robbed you of quality and quantity of life, and that of your children, pets, and anyone else you are responsible for feeding. It has dampened your own energy frequency attracting more negative energy, and you have paid for abuse to continue.

You have spent your precious money on condoning a world that is not the most health-giving, contributes to abuse, and is controlled by industries that only want money from you.

Oh, and did I mention it has poisoned you with chemicals and antibiotics?

Considering all these factors, how much of a bargain is that fake chicken, really?

And considering all the health and metaphysical benefits of supporting true food and healthy organic free-range humanly killed chicken, how much value are you getting by spending more and getting the real deal?

**We get what we pay for.**

By buying directly from the farmer who has respected and loved his animals, you are creating a world worth living in again.

## Vegetarians/Vegans:

If you are a vegetarian or vegan, the same applies to the food you buy too.

Energy is energy. All life, plants included, has a frequency and absorb the energies of those responsible for growing them and what's in the soil. You are still what you eat.

Ensure your food is organic where possible.

Soya, tofu, sweeteners and palm oil are widely used in vegan products, which have a seriously negative energy impact, and not good for health.

So if you do not eat meat, then don't think you are healthier unless you are aware of the ingredients and energy negativity value of the ingredients. If you still eat dairy and eggs, then it is crucial you buy only the organic happiest possible, bearing in my mind that dairy and eggs, even the good ones, are still acidic forming.

**Note:** most soya products are grown with genetically modified beans (GM or GMO) and that is **bad news**. If a product does not state clearly on the packaging that it is NON-GMO then it probably isn't. Truly organic, and Non-GMO are huge selling points so manufacturers will want to advertise this clearly to win more customers.

I **boycott palm oil** and it angers me that it is in so many products. The only reason is that it is cheap to manufacture, yet there are plenty of alternatives such as olive oil, coconut oil or sunflower oil to use instead.

So if you are a vegetarian or a vegan mainly because of animal rights, then you are going against your principles by buying dairy or palm oil.

Palm oil production affects the rainforests, Orangutans and other wild habitats.

Humans are so bloody selfish at times. When are we going to live with nature, not against it? When I say I boycott it, I mean it, even when it does not suit me. I was looking for some nut butter without sugar and I found an organic hazelnut butter but the other ingredient was palm oil. I would rather go without than fund that industry, so I put it back on the shelf. There was no nut butter I could buy that did not have either sugar or palm oil in it, and yet those ingredients are not necessary.

The week after I was in Sedona (US) and in the shop I came across locally home-made hazelnut butter made with 100% organic nuts grown lovingly (no GMO) and packaged in a glass jar with a planet-friendly label and there was only one ingredient: Organic Hazelnuts. It needs to be kept in the fridge but has a long sell-by date. It cost $25, so about twice the price of the organic one with the palm oil, but I made the decision that the world changes one purchase at a time.

I wasn't going to compromise my values to save a few bucks, and it is super tasty.

## Obesity Interlude:

If you suffer from weight-gain just know it is not really your fault, it has nothing to do with willpower.

It is mainly due to manufacturers adding hidden sugars and sweeteners (if they don't try to hide this fact why are there over 50 names for sugar!) to make us eat more.

Sweeteners muck about with our hormones. Sugar with our energy levels.

It is partly due to their marketing campaigns brainwashing us with images and adverts of what to eat.

It has a lot to do with the quality of food we now have.

We are undernourished. Our bodies do not get adequate nutrients and good energy from the food we eat, even food we cook ourselves, as regular fruit, vegetables and meat are laden with antibiotics, pesticides, fungicides, chemicals and our soil is lacking in selenium and copper and other good stuff we require.

So we eat volumes but are still hungry and our bodies are still in need of nutrients, so it tries to help by sending out signals in the form of hunger and cravings, but we then snack on the wrong foods.

Our body ignores the non-food storing it as fat and keeps asking for *real* food.

Have you ever noticed that if you have a week or two of just organic food, and no sugar or carbs, or sodas, so just green juices, soups, nuts, plenty of clean water, then you actually eat a lot less and don't get hungry?

One of the most effective ways of losing weight is to eat human-friendly food.

That means organic, fresh, grass-fed/grass-finished happy meat, and with plenty of good water and organic herbal teas. And avoid sugars, commercial food, sodas, coffee, sweeteners and cheap meats or fish.

Also to clear toxins with walks in nature and taking deep cleansing breaths.

If you accompany that with some movement, not necessarily strenuous exercise, then it will really help shift toxins.

Once the toxins are out of the way, the body can deal with the trapped fat.

Being aware of exactly what we eat and where that food came from and the energetic value of it, may help us release excess weight too.

So yes, it is more expensive, but the benefits far outweigh the financial cost.

And if we only, or mainly eat healthy food, then we will need less of it as our bodies will be fed correctly and satisfied with less amount, so in the long run, we save money that way too. And there is no price on feeling good in your body and being slimmer, if you have experience at being overweight then you understand. It sucks, right?

**Make a choice now**: YOU come first, in every decision you make about buying food. YOU come first, then the planet, environment, and rip yourself away from being under the control of food manufacturers, their marketing campaigns or government recommendations.

Deal?

Coolio.

*Make a note in your journal stating that from now on, You, yes you come first and you decide what you spend your money on and what food you buy and eat.*

Interlude over.

* * *

I know this is deep and perhaps too much in this bladder book, but I wish to impart how important it is what food and drink we put in our bodies and why.

To put your bladder health back in your hands, it is important to know where others control it. The food industry, the marketing industry, and government lobbyists are sometimes in control of what you eat. You and only you can now change that.

Shop sensibly and do some research of your own. It is getting easier to source high-quality food now.

Yes, it may cost you more money, but you get what you pay for.

Do you not deserve real food?

Of course, you do, health first, bladder first, that is the A-Team choice.

If you truly cannot afford organic in all that you eat, then compromise, have some organic and some not. Avoid as much added sugar or dairy as possible or better still, chuck them out of your existence. Analyse your food choices, there are still better choices to be made that will help your health.

Remember, the A-Game is to make changes, but even if you just do some of them, it will make a difference. Don't be overwhelmed, commit to making some changes you can easily stick to and do them, then change some more, until you have a nutritional **A-Team** that you can live with.

**Say YES to:**

Organic vegetables in quantity, quality and variety. They all have different fibres and nutrients and our gut loves the mix as it keeps all the good guys happy and the candida at bay. Ensure to buy organic where possible in all foods.

- Green vegetables
- Healthy oils (Olive, Coconut, Avocado, Walnut, Sunflower)
- Avocado
- Organic Apple Cider Vinegar (with the mother)
- Lemons
- Garlic
- Onions
- Ginger
- Turmeric
- Cinnamon
- Herbs
- Chamomile, mint, nettles…
- Aloe Vera (high quality using the gel as the first ingredient, not the leaf)
- Some fruit (we can have some but not daily, and due to its nature, it needs to be eaten on an empty stomach so it passes through quickly in your tract, and seasonally is best)
- Spring or mineral water (annoyingly, most come in plastic bottles but it is still preferable to unfiltered tap water)
- Redbush Tea (rooibos)
- Hibiscus
- Rosehip

Some say that vitamin C may help keep urine acidic and acid will help kill certain bacteria. That said urine is supposed to be PH neutral and it is the neutrality that is most effective at keeping germs at bay.

It is difficult for a body to get diseases if it has a perfectly balanced PH or slightly alkaline.

You should get plenty of Vitamin C if you are following the nutritional protocol, but providing you source a healthy non-sugar, non-chemical supplement, then adding Vitamin C supplements may help. I also suggest Vitamin D, Vitamin K and Magnesium supplements especially in the winter but always check doses with a natural health professional.

This may help to ensure adequate bone strength as when our food is too acidic, the body regulates the PH level by using minerals and calcium to dilute the acid, the most readily available is in our bones.

This is where ensuring an **A-Team** in nutrition will help.

I sometimes reduce the acidity in my body by drinking alkaline and the quickest way is diluting food-grade bicarbonate of soda in water. I use a 1 teaspoon in a glass of water and have it on an empty stomach or right before bed.

The original bladder health program that I designed for myself was for 8 weeks. I have now changed the program into protocols to follow daily.

**Bladder health and the protocols are a lifestyle, not a fad or diet.**

If you have suffered from chronic cystitis for some time, stick with all the protocols, or at least the nutrition, toilet, and sexual protocols for at least 8 weeks, to clear out candida and give your whole system a rest from inflammatory foods and behaviours. Then, you can reintroduce things slowly and see where your tolerance levels are. **Everyone's Bladder A-Team will look different.**

Before I started this program, I got to the point that I couldn't even have some sweet chilli sauce with my chicken, or a teaspoon of honey, because the candida in my bladder, and probably in my gut, was so rife that any more sugar would be too invasive, so I had to be very strict. You need to starve it completely. Even if you feel better before 8 weeks, keep going, your bladder will be grateful.

The more you put into your regime now, the more your bladder will be tolerable for the occasional slip later.

When you do have some inflammatory food, then drink plenty to flush it out, the quicker it is out of your system, the better. We don't want it lurking too long soaking your bladder walls.

There are ways of having a happy fun life and a happy bladder, it is about using common sense, but we can only enjoy common sense when we know why we get cystitis and how to balance out the things that could trigger it.

Sadly, at the moment at least, sense is not all that common in the world of cystitis.

Now you have your protocols, train yourself to tick more from the A-Team and less from the trigger list.

Fasting is useful too. It helps to give your whole digestive tract a rest and enables a deep cleanout. When you fast, your body does the spring cleaning, great news to reset candida levels and other imbalances.

Your body will do the work, you just need to stop eating and drink plenty of clean water, hot water with organic lemon, hot water with fresh ginger, organic nettle, peppermint or chamomile teas, and high-quality sugar-free aloe vera gel juice.

Fast from 14 hours up to 3 days, and then slowly introduce bladder-friendly food again. Do this whenever you feel the need to, or after a binge, or maybe once a month. Check with a medical practitioner before fasting as it may not be ideal if you have certain conditions or medication.

Some people enjoy intermittent fasting, allowing your system a break from food for 14 to 18 hours on a daily basis. I do this at times, I eat my last meal in the evening at about 6 pm and then don't eat again until about noon the following day, giving myself 18 hours off food. Some people can't go without breakfast, so this is a personal choice, but it works for me. One reason it does it since the menopause I feel sick in the mornings and don't want to it anyway.

Exercise also helps to clear the blood of sugars and creates endorphins, happy hormones that are always welcome, but they do also cause cortisol and stress hormones. Also, ensure proper daily hygiene protocol after exercise.

There will be a tipping point. Once cleansed and rested, your body may cope with some gluten, dairy, sugars, alcohol, cigarettes, although, the A-Team would be to exterminate those for good, but should you choose for them to still play a part in your life, that is OK as long as you realise they are from the trigger list and ensure to tick more from the A-Team to balance out.

Some days you will want to drink too much alcohol and end up in bed with that bloke you fancied for ages and not bother with the sexual hygiene protocol.

Some days you will forget or can't be bothered to drink enough water and have lots of coffee or wine.

Some days you will have negative self-talk and not love yourself too much.

All this is OK, just be aware of it and counteract when you can. And don't beat yourself up or feel guilty as if you decide to have it, enjoy it and then continue on your health journey.

## Finding Your Fulcrum

The fulcrum is what I call the tipping point, where if you have just one more tick from the trigger list, you have gone too far and your bladder won't cope.

At this point, really listen to your body signals. If this happens, I have created an emergency reset meditation. It is important to do so to help your bladder get rid of inflammation or candida as soon as possible before full-blown cystitis occurs.

If it does occur, go to the doctors to check for infection or any other bladder issue.

**Remember that symptoms for most bladder problems feel the same.**

You are not a failure if you do get cystitis again.

Deep breath, don't allow frustration or self-hatred to creep in.

Connect to your body and think back to what happened to trigger this bout.

Look at the trigger checklist, over the last 48 hours, what did you do, eat, or drink that may have contributed?

This is so that you get used to linking behaviours with cystitis, this is powerful as it reminds you that you are in control and it removes the victimhood.

But don't blame yourself either, take responsibility and bring in your

Bladder A-Team. Put it down to experience and add it to your learning.

## Artificial Sweeteners

I promised earlier that I would elaborate in this section on some detrimental foods, especially the nerve-killers in food and drink, including what we give our kids.

Artificial sweeteners are for many reasons silent killers.

There are many on the market. The following are major generic categories. Each one will have sub-categories too. I won't list them but they include all the syrups, the alcohols, and the branded sweetener names.

The major players are acesulfame potassium, aspartame, cyclamate, glycerol, hydrogenated starch hydrolysate (HSH), isomalt, lactitol, maltitol, including hydrogenated high maltose content glucose syrup, neotame, saccharin, erythritol, sorbitol, sucralose and xylitol.

In my opinion, they are *all* bad but let's concentrate on aspartame. If you wish to research for yourself there is a lot of information on all sweeteners available. I'm using one example to elaborate on the seriousness of what is deemed as food in modern society.

Don't be fooled if advertising says they are made from natural stuff. Remember arsenic and mercury are natural but deadly to humans.

Aspartame was invented in a laboratory. It is made by mixing L-phenylalanine and L-aspartic acid, (amino acids), and methanol together.

L-phenylalanine is mostly derived from the excrement (poo!) of genetically modified bacteria, such as E-Coli. I mean, already you should be hearing warning bells.

It is then cut (like they do with heroin) with different *questionable* fillers. One of those is usually genetically modified corn, which is *seriously* toxic in itself. Other fillers have been exposed to fertilisers, pesticides, fungicides, and monosodium glutamate (MSG).

* * *

MSG is questionable because it causes controversy between some who say it is bad for human health and a neurotoxin, linked to a ridiculous amount of health issues, including urological issues such as prostate swelling, frequent bladder pain, cystitis, vaginal bleeding and swelling, and the frequent need to pee.

Some say, including the FDA, that it is safe. It is used as a food enhancer in mainly Chinese food, soups, and hams.

It is also a naturally occurring substance found in cheese, grapes, mushrooms, tomatoes and other foods. MSG is sodium salt of glutamic acid, a naturally occurring non-essential amino acid.

Scientists originally extracted sodium salt from seaweed. In manufactured products, you may find MSG listed as yeast extract, hydrolysed vegetable protein, HVP, or autolysed protein. It usually is now produced from wheat gluten and sugar beet molasses. So, in my opinion, naturally occurring MSG from seaweed or tomatoes is probably OK, as long as you tolerate it, but manufactured stuff probably isn't, especially if using sugar or gluten.

It is recognised that it is not safe for everyone, as some do have allergies to it, and those that do should also avoid foods where MSG is naturally occurring, such as tomatoes or soy-sauce. So, I shall leave that one up to you. The most important judge of whether MSG (or any food) is OK for you, is your body.

I do have MSG at times, as I will still have Chinese food as it is gorgeous, and I still want it in my life. But that is my choice.

I'm not as lenient with sweeteners, and that is also because I hate the taste of super-sweet and fake-sweet. Yuk. Sweeteners make my tongue recoil.

* * *

So now, back to that white stuff. All these toxic compounds create the white powder called aspartame that is found in an alarming amount of foods and drinks.

Eating it causes further problems. Aspartame forces our body to create a chemical called formaldehyde. This is a highly toxic neuro compound. It is a nerve killer.

Outside our bodies, formaldehyde is also a killer. It is an environmental pollutant used in many things, such as embalming the dead.

Formaldehyde is ranked as one of the most hazardous compounds for humans and can damage the liver, the lungs, the intestines, and the reproductive system.

And if nerve-killing wasn't enough, aspartame also tricks our body to thinking we are ill because artificial aspartic acid crosses the blood-brain barrier, potentially mimicking symptoms of multiple sclerosis, Parkinson's disease, and epilepsy. It is linked to weight gain and diabetes.

It changes the body's natural balance of hormones.

Artificial sweeteners such as aspartame, sucralose, and sorbitol can remain inside your organs for years. Aspartame has been found in children's' brains. A large amount of ingested sweeteners (especially sucralose) will be stored in the liver, kidneys (and hence bladder), and intestines.

Can you see how having artificial sweeteners can affect your urinary tract?

Aspartame's toxic effects are cumulative, building up over time. Don't be fooled that because you feel OK after having some, that it is not killing you slowly.

Every time you consume a drug, food, or drink with artificial sweeteners, you are damaging your nerves and causing yourself serious damage.

Check what is in your children or pet food. Unless it is *truly* free from artificial sweeteners and *not* been in contact with pesticides, fungicides, or insecticides, especially Zyklon B gas, then you are exposing them to some of what was used in gas chambers, even at minute levels, is that still OK with you?

Scientists created nerve-toxins for the Nazis to kill people in camps. They were originally designed as chemical warfare, for genocide. Since then, someone decided it was OK to use them in pesticides and additives in food and drink.

By consuming these we are in effect committing slow suicide. Enough said.

The only sweetener that I consider natural is *organic* fruit (not fructose as a powder but actual fruits, and the leaves from the plant Stevia, not the white powder they make from it) and maybe raw organic honey, although this is not a natural state as bees processed it from pollen, but it isn't a process that harms human health, unless the honey's been heated or treated with nasties, and a lot of honey has. Pure organic raw maple syrup is also natural but finding one that has not been processed is hard.

Aspartame, high-fructose corn syrup (HFCS), and all sweeteners really are nasty pieces of work.

OK, I hear you ask, why then is it permitted by the governments?

*Really?*

Governments don't always know what is bad for us until enough people have died from it. This takes decades to prove. In the meantime, questionable items are approved. This is to profit pharmaceuticals and the food and drink industries.

**Note:** I'm not picking on any brand here per se, but I'm using *Coca-Cola* as an example as this information is widely available on the internet and so I'm not exactly divulging anything new or secret. I'm also not boycotting them or any brand as they have a right to make business, but I am using their story as an example of what I mean about not relying on governments.

Coca-Cola was originally made with cocaine and caffeine. Hence its name, *Coca* for cocaine and *Cola* for kola nut caffeine. When it came out, the government did *not* acknowledge that cocaine was bad for human health. They also didn't see a problem with caffeine, tobacco or opium. Drinking Coca-Cola, smoking and getting doped up was supposedly fine.

Cigarettes contain deadly nasties and look how long it took for governments to tell us. And they *still* haven't made smoking illegal! Anyone over 16 can buy and use cigarettes anywhere. And yet this is what they contain: tobacco, formaldehyde, (yep that nasty bastard) pesticides (so nerve-gas), fibreglass (in the filter), aluminium, and other heavy metal toxins.

**Note:** mercury and formaldehyde are two of the most deadly neurotoxins known to medical science.

If you are still unsure of how these substances affect our health, research it. Or just trust me: they are *seriously* bad news.

Once cocaine was deemed toxic, it was named an illegal substance. Coca-Cola was forced to remove the *coke* from their product. Cocaine is addictive, so to ensure the drink was still going to be purchased by the masses, Coca-Cola replaced cocaine with a legal narcotic giving a similar addiction. They replaced cocaine with sugar.

In recent years, now that finally the government was forced to admit that sugar is problematic, companies use an alternative. In the last 25 years or so, they also use artificial sweeteners, aspartame being the most well-known.

We have moved from cocaine to sugar to artificial sweeteners.

All are toxic and yet two of those are *natural.*

How long before aspartame and other artificial toxins are finally classed as too toxic for human consumption and deemed illegal substances?

Then guess what the drink, food, and drug companies will use to continue selling their legal poisons? Well, it will be a new lab-created substance that will damage our health until it is finally declared not fit for human consumption.

**Are you really willing to wait until some government finally tells you that aspartame is bad for you before you stop consuming it or giving it to your children and pets?**

*You* decide what is good for you.

*You* decide what you eat and drink.

Do not leave this important decision to governments.

\* \* \*

## Dairy

I promised you earlier that I would elaborate on why dairy is so detrimental, so let's conclude this section with that.

All dairy is inflammatory, it is acidic forming non-food and causes inflammation/swelling throughout our body. Some people tolerate it more than others, but it still doesn't make it a food fit for any human.

Female mammals (including women) create milk to feed their new-born and toddler. That is it. The only time humans should be having milk is as new-borns and as toddlers up to about two years old. The only milk we should be having then is from our mother, or from another human woman. So, milk from our own species, that's it.

Beyond that age, milk is no longer necessary, so let's say once you have all your baby teeth, also known as *milk* teeth, again the clue is in our language, you have everything you need from your mother's milk.

That's it, bye-bye milk, forever. That is natural, it is how we were designed.

No other mammal deliberately drinks milk from another species and not beyond the formative baby stage either.

Yet, *somehow*, most of us have decided it is perfectly OK to drink milk as adults and to drink milk from other species.

Er, hello?

Each species is different. We cannot digest or use the goodness in other species' milk because we are not designed to. The only being that has any business drinking cow's milk is a calf. That's it. It's simple logic.

Yet, somehow, the dairy industry and their government lobbyists brainwash us to think that we need milk, cheese, yoghurt, or butter, for our health and bones.

*Really?*

Who profits from that lie?

Not you, not your teeth, not your bones, not your bladder, and certainly not the cows.

Dairy is so acidic that our stomach needs to dilute it using potent alkaline, calcium. The best source it will find is in your bones. So every time you have dairy, instead of adding calcium into your body, you take it from your own skeletal system.

Yep, read that bit again.

Dairy, in my opinion, *contributes* to osteoporosis, chronic cystitis, weakened bones, weakened teeth, sinus issues, asthma, weakened immune system, any '–itis' condition, and stunted growth.

It does not contribute to human health but damages it, a lot.

It doesn't matter how much calcium and goodness is proven to be in milk (because it is rich and nutritious, for baby cows), we humans are unable to use that goodness as it is not bio-available to our system as we are not designed to have it.

Am I being clear enough here? I know this section is pushing buttons in some of you, just keep going, OK?

We can, however, use up all that lovely goodness from our own mother's breast milk, but not milk from a cow's teat, or any other animal.

No, substituting cow dairy for goat or sheep dairy is not the answer. Using soya milk is not the answer either. How about ditching all dairy, that's the truest answer.

That is the chemical reason why to avoid milk and all dairy.

**Here is another huge factor: energy frequency.**

Energy begets similar energy. The law of attraction.

Remember the basic metaphysics we have already explored...

Now, this isn't true of all the dairy industry, there are still some farmers who love their cows, who feed them organic grass and provide plenty of pastures to roam in, and who milk them lovingly by hand. I found such farms that commercially make their products easily available (in England) during my research, but these are, sadly, rare. There are more of these in rural areas of Europe and the large plains in the US, but the milk we buy in supermarkets mostly don't originate from those.

For the most part, milk comes from *seriously* abused cows.

Cows have feelings: they experience love and loss as all mammals do.

Imagine giving birth, then having your baby ripped away from you, hearing its desperate cries.

Then whilst heart-broken, devastated and grieving, you are hooked up to a seriously painful milking machine and pumped for ages each day until you are dried up.

Then you are artificially impregnated again and go through the grief cycle over and over for years.

During that time your nipples get blocked, your breasts swell up with puss, they hurt to touch, and yet, no one cares, you are still plugged into the milking machine, relentlessly.

Everyone is ignoring your cries, agony, broken-heart and damaged soul, because all they want is your milk, as cheaply as possible, to sell it to humans who don't need it.

Let's not even mention what happens to the baby cow that milk was made for. You can fill in those blanks, and yes, the calf's energy frequency is still linked to their mother's milk, even if they didn't get any, and so it does end up in the end-product that ends up in you, and your children, and your pets.

Back to that dairy cow, after years of constant abuse, agony, grief, losing countless children, being stuck in a pen, and treated worse than any vicious criminal, you die a painful death, your carcass disposed of without thought or care. That's it, your life is over, and it comes as a relief. Then another young cow takes your tiny pen, forced to stand in old manure and puss, and the process continues, endlessly.

All that so humans can poison themselves with milk in their gluten cereals that all contribute to chronic bad health.

So, all the misery that went into producing your pint of milk is going inside you.

It is the building block you are giving your body to create its new cells with the very cells that decide your current state, the health of your future and your life-span.

Is that milk in your coffee or that cheese on toast *really* worth all that?

So, now you know. Every time you buy dairy unless it specifies 'truly organic, from happy cows and no cow or calf was harmed to make this product', then, you are willingly contributing to one of the worst industries for animal abuse.

And every time you eat dairy, you are knowingly most probably ingesting the energy frequency of agony, grief, puss, loss and pure misery.

**Please, if not for the cows, then for your own bladder's health, do consider giving up dairy, or at least reducing the amount you consume.**

I did warn you that I wasn't going to shy away from truths, that taboos were going to get smashed, and that I was going to do what I could to awaken you.

All of which is my duty as the author to the promised 'fully-functional guide to obliterating all bladder pains'.

If I believe that something can affect your bladder, it will get mentioned in this book.

**As you noted in my introduction, I won't apologise for that: it's my job.**

For me to do my job properly, I have to prise open lots of things that we, as a society and individually, have swept under the carpet (hence into your bladder).

Then, all can be explored and pulled apart, and that gives you your power back because knowledge is key.

If you know tarot, parts of this book will act as the 'tower card', tearing down structures, belief systems, and society's damaging ways, to clear the ground, and start fresh. It may hurt, but it is worth it. Fortune favours the brave.

Open your eyes and change your world by making truer choices.

So now, if you choose to buy dairy, at least you do it with your eyes wide open, and that then makes it your true choice. You are no longer controlled by profit-hungry industries or misleading food pyramids.

The dairy and grains section should be deleted.

It doesn't lessen the detrimental chemical or energetic impact of eating dairy, but it gives you the freedom to know exactly what your money is condoning.

**The Bladder A-Team** does not eat any dairy or sweeteners and scrutinises food labels. Unfortunately, like sugar, milk, whey or casein sneak into lots of products.

If you can't do without milk, then the best alternative is organic non-GMO almond or other nut milk. You can make your own by whizzing up organic raw nuts with mineral water. Another good alternative is organic coconut milk, or organic coconut yoghurts without added sugars, sweeteners, or colourings.

Being awake means freedom. So it's OK if you decide that you still want cow dairy products, but please, do yourself a favour, and pay more for buying some as organically and ethically produced as possible.

I share a link in the *Products & Services Reference* brand that, in my opinion, is as humane as possible for commercially produced milk. There will still be low energy links due to the loss of calves and being milked, but less than the mass-produced milk brands or cheaper milk in supermarkets.

Also, the taste will be so much nicer and richer coming from organic grass-fed happier cows. So if you want cow dairy, then this is a solution. Do be aware that, chemically, milk is still detrimental to our health, even if it is organic and from happier cows or from A2 producing cows such as Jersey. Some think this milk is easier to digest, but it is still detrimental in every way.

The choice is yours. I have made you aware, so now my job in terms of nutritional protocols is done.

I share what food and drink I have in the Products & Services Reference.

* * *

A-Team nutrition is to eat and drink foods that nature made, not man.

Eat food closest to its most natural state and of course, wild, organic, non-GMO, ethically traded, and that is safe and designed for human consumption, by nature.

Choose 'happy energy' food where possible.

I'm not concerned about calories in food and drink, only the quality and naturalness of those calories. Your body can handle real calories as it is classed as fuel, so it will use it or ditch it.

It will suffer from fake calories, as they are not real fuel and the body will feel the need to store these, wrap them up in fat and water, and hide them in fat-cells, out of harm's way.

**Do not fear high-quality real fuel calories, fear the fake.**

**Example:** eat as much organic avocado mashed in organic extra virgin olive oil spread on home-made organic paleo nut bread and enjoy it (real fuel). Avoid butter, margarine, or low-fat spreads on gluten bread (fake fuel).

Remember if we give our bodies real food then it will want less as it is nutritious and so we should not put on weight by eating good food, providing we don't overeat or mix it with rubbish.

Remember that what is classed as food nowadays is mostly not real fuel for humans.

## 8- Hydration Protocol

Start the day with a large glass of room temperature water. Then have hot water with a slice of organic freshly cut lemon and/or a slice of freshly cut ginger or a couple of tablespoons of organic apple cider vinegar.

Have aloe vera gel juice, either that you make yourself with organic aloe vera, using the fleshy gel inside, or ready-made from a reputable company.

**Note**: the A-Team would gulp first thing in the morning to hydrate fast, and then sip water during the day so not to overload, not down the two litres of water in one go in the evening because you forgot to drink it during the day. That being said, it is better to do that than not drink it at all. Aim for a minimum of 2 litres of water per day.

Drink water at room temperature or warm, but not cold. Avoid putting ice in your drinks or keeping water in the fridge. Cold drinks are not good for the bladder.

The body prefers body-temperature water or at least room temperature so it can take it straight to the cells, if it is too cold it needs to spend calories warming it up and will most likely just get rid of the water faster than desired.

Sip between 1.5 and 5 litres of mineral, spring still water, or filtered tap water during the day. The amount you need will depend on your size and lifestyle.

You need more than 1.5 litres if you are bigger (in mass)and heavier (in weight) than average, live or holiday in hot climates, sunbathing, exercising, have sex that day, ill or feverish, tired, if your diet includes lots of non-foods or non-organic, if you smoke, travelling or in air-conditioning a lot, or if you are still thirsty.

If I'm combatting a UTI or candida cystitis, I will be drinking almost continuously to flush out the germ or yeast. The one exception is the cramping or 'overactive cystitis' where for a few hours I don't drink at all to give it a chance to reset, but even then, I still aim for 2 litres.

**Note**: there is a maximum amount of water our bodies can cope within a day but this is usually set high, and most people suffer from not having enough water, rather than having too much. If you are concerned ask your medical practitioner.

When I have really bad infection cystitis, I have been known to drink over 8 litres of water in a day and be OK.

The only time I was a bit dodgy and felt over-watered was during a really bad bacterial cystitis and wanted to dislodge the germ from the bladder wall and pee it out asap, so I gulped a 5-litre bottle in one go (and nearly threw up), and then slowly downed another, whilst waiting for the doctor appointment.

Three hours later when he dipped my urine, he was shocked to see it was 100% clear, it looked like water, although he still detected blood and infection.

He was pleased that I was drinking plenty, but when I told him I had already 10 litres that day, and it was only lunchtime, he warned me that was far too much and I could harm myself with that amount.

I had not heard of over-hydration before so I looked into it, and agreed.

I did feel some symptoms of over-watering, light-headed, nauseated, and weakened, but it went away after a few hours and it did help to flush out the germ quicker.

**Note**: If you are concerned then do not drink too much in one go or more than 2 litres per day until you ask your medical practitioner for advice.

Increase hydration during the day with your nutrition too. Have high-water content food in your meals such as smoothies, salads, cucumber, home-made soups, celery, melons, and juicy fruits, but fruit only on an empty stomach and not followed by other foods and only when in season.

If you fancy a hot drink, go for a red-bush tea instead of regular black or green teas to avoid caffeine content.

You can try organic herbal teas that are naturally caffeine-free (chamomile, nettle, mint, ginger, lemon and ginger, cinnamon…), there are plenty of choices, ensure to get organic when you can, as teas do get sprayed a lot with chemicals.

Don't bother with decaffeinated tea and coffee unless it specifies 'naturally decaffeinated', as the process to remove caffeine is laden with chemicals unless it has been purely sun-dried, which is more expensive and therefore rarer.

Obviously, if you are drinking out, then the choice is limited. I do enjoy a nice Earl Grey in cafes, but I have it with almond or soya milk, as I refuse to participate in dairy, and OK that milk may not be unsweetened or no- GM, but at least I am engaging in damage limitation.

You can also have green tea or black tea but where possible buy organic and limit those as caffeine is an irritant to our digestive tract and bladder walls, but you may get away with some if you feel you want to, depending on your personal fulcrum.

If you are a regular coffee with milk and sugar person, that is 3 trigger boxes right there in a cup. Massively inflammatory foods: dairy, sugar and caffeine.

Find an alternative drink, and if you can't because you love your coffee too much, question if it is true love or the control of addictive chemicals and the world of advertising bombarding you with images of what they want you to like and spend your money on. Any addiction is counter-productive to health.

Avoid caffeine, any drink decaffeinated via chemicals, milk, alcohol, sugary drinks, fizzy drinks, yoghurt drinks, sports energy drinks, carbonated water, GMO or sweetened soya milk, squash/cordial, no matter how diluted, flavoured waters and limit any black or green tea.

**Hydrating Our Skin**

Keep your skin well hydrated too, but not with nasty products such as polymers or alcohol and not daily, as the skin needs to breathe and sweat. It needs to be clean and preferably not covered in too much clothing so it can breathe, yes, our skin does breathe, it is another way our body gets rid of toxins.

Moisturise on days where it is hot, or you have sweated a lot, or you came into contact with chemicals, then do protect it.

If you are going swimming in a public pool laden with chemicals and chlorine, and this is good as it kills off the germs, but it is bad for our skin and hydration levels, and an irritant to our precious holes.

The best swimming pools are those with ozonated water or salt.

What I do, where possible, is swim in the ocean, lakes, or rivers, so in natural waters, but when I go to a Jacuzzi or a chemically swimming pool, I shower first then dry off and lather organic coconut oil or organic olive oil on my skin and hair and inside sinuses, so that all my skin is covered, including my precious holes, and that way it provides a natural barrier against the harsh chemicals, then I shower again after.

I use primarily 4 moisturisers, either aloe vera gel, propolis cream, organic raw coconut oil, or organic olive oil. It is good to moisturise your skin regularly but not all the time.

Maybe twice a week, have a ritual after bathing (following all hygiene protocols). Massage your whole body and face with your chosen moisturiser and at the same time, apply metaphysical energy by imagining you are sending love or golden light through your hands into your skin, and smile.

Smiling releases endorphins and helps to be more present and the more present you can be whilst touching your body, the better it will work.

If you have dry skin or exposed to the sun regularly, then moisturising most nights would be ideal, and chose to be in the shade, not the sunlight.

**Skin quality comes from within**. Great nutrition, drinking high-quality aloe vera and plenty of water is what the skin needs. Ensure to keep it happy by using high-quality products on your skin and laundry, anything that touches your skin.

Moisturisation of the skin helps the top layer, but if your diet is bad, you smoke and use commercial products, then moisturising at night isn't going to do much. Skin needs the whole package. Beauty comes from within and without, so inside and out.

## 9- Stress Protocol

Stress, at all levels, is bad for our health and linked to certain types of cystitis.

The only 'good' stress is exercising but we still need to counterbalance this stress by doing long deep stretches to release the cortisol and acid build-up, drink plenty of water to rehydrate, do some deep breathing to calm the nervous system and send a signal that the stress is over and we are safe.

For a happy bladder, we need to reduce stress levels. In this world, we are bombarded with stress triggers. Find out what makes you stressed and counteract it.

Build up an anti-stress routine and increase deep relaxing activities in your life.

**Enjoy some of these on a regular basis:**

- massages
- holistic therapies
- yoga
- exercising
- martial arts
- health retreats
- personal development workshops
- chi-gong
- tai-chi
- meditations
- music, playing it, listening to it or writing it
- sounds of nature
- going for walks in nature
- being by the sea
- swimming in natural (clean) waters
- painting
- writing

- singing
- chanting
- doodling
- colouring in
- playing an instrument
- napping
- hugging an animal
- talking to a plant
- hugging a tree (yep, why not),
- counselling sessions
- going for a meal with a best friend
- watching a funny film
- reading
- going on holiday
- making love (following the 'sexual protocol') with a partner you adore

There are so many stress-relieving methods that you will definitely resonate with some. The list above just touches on some of them to get you started in thinking about what is out there.

*Write down in your journal any stress-relief activities you are going to try.*

The more you do them, the more you will allow stress to leave your body.

When possible, avoid your known stress factors, they can come in different forms, for example: certain foods that make you cranky (gluten, sugar, dairy, snacks); that family member that gets you fired up; that boss that makes your skin crawl; listening to the news; reading the newspapers; being with a negative person who moans too much; being around drama-queens; being around piss-takers or bullies; leaving your tax returns to the last minute; shopping during busy times; talking in public; stuck in traffic; in a cramped train, or overspending on credit cards.

When we are stressed, we create adrenaline and cortisol in our body and we become too acidic. Our bodies have to deal with stress at all levels including chemically. This creates an inflamed environment and our muscles and organs crease up under the strain. On a chronic basis, is problematic for all of us, but also to our bladder.

The more acid and stress-toxins are in our blood, the more end up in our urine, hence soaking our bladder walls.

So, do anything to bring down your stress levels, pulse, and breathing rate.

A quick effective way to achieve this is to breathe consciously. So, every day, commit to a routine of taking 5 (or any number) of deep breaths, being present in your body. Breathe in and hold your breath allowing it to get deep into your cells then breathe out. Remember to get up, stretch and breathe with intention several times during the day. This is a mini-holiday for your body and mind.

Meditation is important for good health. Try it. Why not? There are so many free tutorials to download from the Internet. Experience several types to see which ones you like best.

There are sounds of nature, guided visualisations, breathing ones, music ones, chanting ones, silent ones, all sorts.

I have created meditations, especially for this book (see the meditation chapter).

If you have not meditated or experienced many holistic therapies before, please don't worry, there are so many available, and if done regularly, you should feel the benefit.

Meditations are not woo-woo or new-age-bullshit, they are a proven method to bring down stress.

## 10- Clear Space Protocol

Your outer environment reflects your inner space and vice versa.

What I like to call: *as within, so without.*

Decluttering is a huge part of health. If surrounded by junk, your thoughts will turn to junk and your body will get stressed. Energy begets similar energy, remember?

Declutter at all levels. The freer on the outside, the freer you will be inside.

This includes social decluttering.

Oh, yes, you know what I mean: that friend who rings you every time she is troubled, but is not there when you need to talk; the one that always wants help, or who rings you when most inconvenient; that other friend who's not really present with you, but uses you; that person is clearly a piss-taker; the boss who treats you like crap; the boyfriend that talks you down…

It's time to let them all go. To have a happy bladder, we need to consider getting rid of people and activities that negatively affect us, or at least create a coping mechanism around them, so they no longer get to us as much.

You will be better off without these fake or disconnected people in your energy field. Remember piss-takers, abusers, controllers, closed-minded people, rule-makers and bullies, all vibrate at low frequencies that could be stored in your bladder.

## Decluttering means removing irritants and junk from your life, from all levels.

Consider each level. Do you have any junk, depressing energies, things or people that no longer serve you well?

**Environmental**: personal space, home, work, closets, clothing, products, books, quality of air, neighbourhood, housemates.

**Social**: people, sports, friends, colleagues, acquaintances, family, news, radio, TV, mode of transport, social media, emails, computer files, hobbies, flirting, dating, sexual partners.

**Mental**: bad thoughts, overthinking, negative belief patterns, other people's opinions, your self-talk, dreams, nightmares, quality of REM sleep.

**Emotional**: blocked or trapped emotions, memories, taboos, secrets that gnaw at you, not-talked-about sexual abuse, bullying, being with the wrong partner, self-sabotage, grief, anger, pissed-off-ness, how you view yourself, self-love issues.

**Spiritual**: following someone else's faith, extremes, religions, rules, past-lives.

**Physical**: your body (inside and out), tattoos, posture, skin, food, hydration, pooing, weeing, sweating, what you eat, drink, touch, smell, hear, taste, see, what is activating your senses, exercise, clothing, washing, massages, sex, masturbation, contact-sport.

**Why media sucks**

The News, *really?* Why do you need to know what journalists or newsreaders want to tell you? The reports are hardly ever true, as in not all sides of a story are told, and usually based on fear-mongering or trying to manipulate you to part with money or power. Have you noticed how charity adverts have this depressing music in the background to activate your sympathetic low side, how newsreaders have a monotone and serious voice…

I gave up reading news, watching the news, or listening to news years ago, and I feel great because of it. If I want to find out what is happening in the world, I can go and research specific issues, I don't need to be bombarded by what's happening elsewhere. How about concentrating on our own lives before focusing on others?

If you can't give it up, if you are addicted to the morning paper, or watching the news on TV, then, just go on a 'media/news holiday' for a while at least.

Whatever frequency is dampening your personal space, find a way to move away from it, or if you can't, then to counteract the effects.

*Write down in your journal all the stuff that is cluttering all your levels and how you plan on reducing those negative influences?*

## 11- Metaphysical Protocol

Oh, wow, here is a deep rabbit hole.

I could wander here for days as it is such a delight for me and an endless topic.

So I will keep it brief and relative to bladder health.

I have written a book on basic metaphysics for those who are more interested, it is not published yet but look out for it on my website or social pages: **www.drjmeyer.com** or **@drjennifermeyer**

So, let's remember that all metaphysics means is beyond physics or beyond the physical/visible realm.

We can see metaphysics as a vast umbrella that is covering a wide spread of topics.

**Topics that at some point have come under the umbrella of metaphysics:**

- Alternative therapies
- Paranormal activities or studies
- personal development
- natural remedies
- foraging
- tree-hugging
- UFO's
- crystals
- essential oils
- oracle and tarot cards
- divination
- numerology
- astrology
- pendulums
- elementals
- mediumship
- psychic readings
- telepathy
- religions

- faith
- energy
- frequencies
- Einstein, Tesla and other vanguard metaphysicians or scientists
- time and space
- law of attraction
- natural laws
- dreams and interpretation
- shamanism
- meditation
- reiki
- quantum physics
- time travel
- sacred geometry
- psychic analysis
- Déja-Vu
- premonitions,
- visions
- creative ideas
- coaching
- healing
- praying
- manifesting
- aliens
- fairies
- elementals
- mythical creatures
- mythology
- magic
- alchemy

- chakras
- auras
- the Clair-senses (clairvoyance, clairaudience, claircognizance, clairsentience, clairgustance, clairsalience, clairempathy)
- ghosts
- spirits
- New-Age
- witches
- demons
- the devil
- God
- paganism
- Wicca
- the unexplainable
- Feng-Shui
- and many, many more.

Some of these are now considered natural, such as crystals and oils, but when I was studying, they were considered metaphysical, woo-woo, or airy-fairy.

Some are cross-overs, adopted by physics and metaphysics, such as Einstein and Tesla who are famous metaphysicians who pushed limits and made the impossible, possible. So, it passes from metaphysical or woo- woo to physical and science.

Science is a way for humans to explain things. Gravity always existed, even before it was 'discovered' by man and explained in a tangible way. Gravity itself doesn't care if it is considered science or magic, it just exists. It's man who is obsessed with proving stuff and classing things right or wrong, black or white. Duality is a man-made thing.

Before scientists invented the microscope, we had no idea that germs, microbes or anything smaller than what we could see, existed, and anyone talking about their possible existence would have been ridiculed, and the matter would have been classed as metaphysics at best and insanity at worst. Then, when a scientist invented such an instrument and could prove the existence of microbes, it passed to science and became fact.

So, when man finally invents a tool that can see fairies, they too will pass from metaphysics to science.

We, our bodies, are the most advanced tools on the planet. We need to re-learn how to use them properly.

Why wait until someone invents tools to believe in what you know, somewhere within you, to be true?

Metaphysics isn't just faith, it is an inner knowing that goes beyond the present ability of science.

### I see metaphysics as the ability to bring magic to everyday life.

A man once took offence to the word *energy* during a talk I did and proclaimed angrily that energy is a science word and it means a light bulb going on, it is an energy we can see.

How limiting is that belief?

The energy existed before man invented a lightbulb and how to harness electricity. Worlds change as do belief systems and we are now in an abundant time where metaphysics is widely available and no longer taboo, so enjoy it, explore.

When I started studying metaphysics, I was 13 years old. I enquired at libraries and other places where I could study by correspondence and send off for courses in several subjects. I think my first one was a diploma course in the paranormal, and it went on from there.

At 15, I joined a meditation and paranormal class. Once a week we would meet and learn about reading auras, healing chakras, doing different meditations, and we would practice hands-on-healing, telepathy, past-life regression, dream analysis, colour therapy, oils, crystals, and reading tarot cards.

This was hush-hush and I used to call it my 'relaxation class', as back then, these practices were laughed at or you were considered to be 'one of them' and accused of not living in the 'real world'.

I don't agree with that saying, because whatever your life, it is your real world.

We all live on the same planet, but in different worlds.

## Taboo Breaking Interlude:

People who say things like 'you don't live in the real world' or 'grow up', or 'you have no idea about reality', are the closed-minded ones who believe it's their way or no way. These people when challenged will usually reply 'it just is', or 'that's the way things are,' 'or that is how normal people react', or my favourite 'oh that's different', that is when you point out they have double standards.

They think that if you do not act in the same way they do, or react to things how they expect you to, or don't conform to someone else's rules or traditions, then you are defected, arrogant, or immature.

Live in the world you create and are happiest in, and that is no one else's business and their opinion plays no part in your life.

\* \* \*

Back when I started, and for many years to follow, there was no Internet, no Amazon, no Facebook private groups, no Google, no YouTube and no podcasts.

How did we survive? :o)

There were very few magical shops where I could get my tools, tarot cards were hard to come by, and oracle cards were non-existent. But as I was fascinated, my frequency-matched my inner to outer, and I found masters to teach me, clandestine classes, tarot cards, and keen people to group up with, and plenty of correspondence courses and library books on such matters. My journey began and it hasn't stopped.

All humans have the ability to use their senses beyond the physical, we have just forgotten or been forbidden by those wanting control, such as religions and governments.

My grandmother used to read tarot cards and when the priest would visit, she would hide them as it was against their religion. We have been shackled by governments, laws, and religions for aeons. It's time to break free.

Luckily in the 30+ years that I have been studying and practising metaphysics, it has now become more of a norm. I can now buy any tarot or oracle deck, google dream meanings, and information is readily available, especially on the Internet.

Most towns have a New Age shop, and I can talk about metaphysical or quantum physics stuff without fear, and most people will understand and probably have their own oracle cards and metaphysical way of life that is now accepted as the norm.

So that's enough for now, as this book is about bladders, but I did promise you it could also be life-changing if you applied all the protocols, and metaphysics is powerful, so it did need to be at least mentioned here, enough to pique your interest to embark on your own metaphysical adventure. I'd be happy to hold your hand on that journey too when the time is right and we meet in another book.

*For now, though, back to the bladder.*

## Specific metaphysical tools to help the bladder:

**Crystals:** carnelian, ruby, orange, red or brown agate, black tourmaline, onyx, blue crystals vibrating to water or healing. Crystals relating to the first and second chakras. Use these to meditate with or massage your tummy and lower back with, or put in your bath, or have a crystal reiki healing session with them.

**Chakras:** the first and second. The root (red) located at feet/legs and groin area, and the sacral (orange) located in the lower abdomen, lower back, pelvic and bladder area. Massage or meditate on these areas and send loving energy to ensure they are clear and strong.

**Colours:** red, orange, brown, black, and blue. Colour therapy, or wearing these colours, or meditating with them in mind.

**Elements:** water, for waterworks and emotional healing. Water is the main element of urine and the bladder is a water-bag. Fire as the sacral chakra is about creativity and joy and fire is the element of creation and passion. Use these elements as visionaries in meditations.

* **Elementals:** I did say earlier that I would elaborate a little in this section about water elementals and why they are linked to our waterworks. We all live on Earth and our bodies come from nature, so we are connected to it. There are four main elements that make up this planet and our bodies; fire, earth (metal and wood come under Earth), air, and water. The magic they create when all merged is called the 5th element, called ether, magic, or chi.

The spirits or energy linked to these elements are called elementals. Each element (physical domain) has a metaphysical guardian (elemental).

The elementals linked to water are sometimes called Undines, Water Sprites, Water Nymphs, or Mermaids. They are the 'beings' or the magic of water.

As we are mainly made of water, this element and elementals are crucial for our survival. The element of water is required for our bodies to live. We drink it to hydrate and stay alive.

We need the essence of water too, its magical counterpart. The elementals help us deal with the metaphysical links to water. These are our emotions, subconscious mind, menstrual cycles, psyche, and our deep dark secrets.

So with our bladders then, the water element helps keep them moist, clean and makes up urine and without it, we would have cystitis all the time and quickly die.

The water elementals help with clearing out stored energies from our bladder leftover from self-belief patterns, abuse, bullying, rape, not feeling worthy, and any feelings of being dried-up, or abandoned.

Water elementals can help bring us fresh water of life at an energy level and help put out any unwanted fires. Unwanted fire issues could be anger, frustration, burning, overwhelmed, over-burdened, burnt-out or deserted, as in left out in the blazing desert.

Call upon the water elementals to help soothe your bladder. Work with them in specific meditations to put out old flames (**in the bladder, not your exes!**) and to help flush out old emotions and blockages.

**Meditations:** more details in the 'Meditation' chapter later.

**Essential Oils:** use diluted in a carrier oil and use for massage, or a few drops (no more than 5) in a bath, or smell them. Ylang-Ylang helps to relieve the urge to pee and relax deeply, particular good for overactive bladders. Clary sage is a mild painkiller. Pumpkin seed oil helps reduce urinary frequency. Lavender oil is anti-spasmodic. And for good measure, orange or bergamot as these are great anti-depressants and pick-me-ups, always useful when dealing with any kind of bladder issue. See the products list for which brand of oils I use and recommend.

**Holistic Treatments:**

Regular massages, especially deep tissue to help drain toxins and encourage a better flow of the lymph system.

Acupuncture, tell your therapist you would like help with your kidneys and bladder. The ancient Chinese understood that our waterworks related to emotions, and so the therapist may work on your heart meridians for bladder issues.

Reiki, crystal reiki, and any hands-on-healing that you trust, including remote healing from therapists afar, or even receiving prayers from well-wishers.

**Herbs**: goldenseal may prevent bacteria clinging to urinary walls. Bearberry leaf and uva ursi reduces inflammation and fights infection. Pau d'arco helps reduce inflammation, especially in the bladder. Nettle soothes the urinary tract and prostate pain. Chamomile is antiseptic, anti-inflammatory and soothing.

Not cranberry juice or tablets. In my opinion, it is a myth that cranberry helps, in my experience, it made it worse. Some people say it helped them, but I think that was a coincidence, as all cystitis has a time-limit where candida or bacteria dies, and then the symptoms will lessen and go away, maybe it was that and not the cranberry that they noticed.

If cranberry juice works well for you, then obviously still use it.

**Magnets:** use either a large magnet or hematite to rub over your bladder with intentions of clearing negative energy and enhancing your aura/personal morphic field. You can place small magnets on your tummy over the bladder with plasters.

## Stored Energies

As I mentioned earlier, in metaphysics everything is related, everything matters and energy begets similar energy, right, still with me? Good.

So, we have a different level of being, the physical being the densest, heaviest, most physical. I like to class them as follows.

See the previous illustration in Part One.

**Physical level**: the body, the environment, this planet, meridians.

**Emotional level**: all emotions, feelings, memories, meridians.

**Mental level**: thoughts, belief systems, dreams, memories, astral travelling.

**Spiritual level**: faith, deep rooted-beliefs about existence, past-life memories, astral travelling and connecting to other frequencies/dimensions, spirits.

**Auric level**: the aura is a bubble of frequencies related connecting all of us together, it also hosts our chakras and surrounds our whole being, and it is morph-able and can change frequencies all the time, like the shields on the *Star Trek Enterprise*.

**Chakras** are energy spheres rotating at different frequencies, we have many of them. The 7 most known are root, sacral, diaphragm, heart, throat, brow, and top of the head. They are bridges for all our levels to connect together. Our organs will be assigned to one or two chakras, and we are all interconnected. The bladder resonates most with the sacral chakra and the root chakra.

Our lower earth chakras energetically connect right down to the centre of the earth and our highest chakras to our soul, or source.

**Meridians** are like tubes of energy running up and down our body and also linked to all levels. The points in them are used by martial artists, acupuncturists and acupressurists and for EFT (Emotional Freedom Tapping).

The chakra system comes from Ayurveda medicine.

The meridian system from ancient Chinese medicine.

See yourself as an entire being, not just your body, but all your levels of existence.

You are truly amazing. Right?

Absolutely.

You rock, girlfriend!

The A-Game metaphysically means understanding the basics to connect all that makes health important. This entails bringing awareness to your energy body (your metaphysical existence) and then applying some protocols such as having holistic treatments, doing regular meditations and conversing with your bladder.

When something has an impact on us, it matters. If our physical body is hurt, say we get hit by a truck, the damage is obvious and we need it fixed, if we didn't die.

Physical trauma is easy enough to spot and fix, usually with the help of the medical world, as they deal mainly, if not entirely, on the physical body level, most do not even acknowledge the existence of our other levels or the chakras or meridians.

So when something impacts us at other levels, what do you think happens?

Correct, the same thing. It hurts and needs to be dealt with, only we don't often acknowledge this and so we sweep it under the carpet or worse, are oblivious to our pain or how to fix it.

We all remember a time when someone said something painful to us, bullied us, made us look stupid. It had an impact; it was like a slap in the face on the emotional or mental level. Had it been a slap in the face at the physical level, we would have applied a soothing cream and stroked it better.

We don't do that for other levels, but we should, and this is why.

Any trauma or impact received will eventually have an effect across all levels. We are interconnected, remember. Anything untreated will cause chronic issues.

Chronic issues will seep into the lower levels.

If the impact was spiritual and unresolved, the energy signature of that incident will cascade into the mental, where we create a belief pattern, a coping mechanism sometimes consciously, sometimes unconsciously. We attract patterns that repeat, which lead to victimhood and the sense of loss of control of our own lives.

If it had a huge impact on us, forced us out of our body, it would have caused health issues at *all* levels.

In terms of the bladder then, let us explore further.

If you were sexually abused as a child or a teenager and this has not been dealt with fully, the energetic impact has dented your emotional, mental, and spiritual bodies at the level of the bladder (as well as other organs).

The energies of a dark secret, feeling powerless, dirty, guilty, shameful, being in pain or feeling a fraud, a liar or a slut, will live inside your bladder.

No, it will not show up on medical scans, but it is there. Eventually, this could have a physical impact and cause cystitis or leave you vulnerable in that area, even though the impact was not on the physical level.

If you wet the bed as a child and were teased or punished for it, it would have caused stress and belief patterns about your waterworks and your ability to control them. You could grow up thinking bladder issues are taboo, creating a vicious circle and a belief pattern that you have bladder or incontinence issues at the physical level, even if the bed-wetting was accidental or due to being scared or not wanting to get up and go to the toilet in the dark.

Any impact at any age will affect our health, but I mentioned as a child or teenager as in that stage of our development, we don't know quite who we are yet and our environment moulds our character and beliefs.

All impacts are just as powerful when we are older, but by then we are already formed by our earlier views of the world and our place within it.

So, as an adult, we not only deal with fresh impacts but also need to dig deep to find the original source of the thing that keeps happening.

To cure the bladder of negative impacts, it is time to be brave and speak out.

Call those toxins and memories to the surface and then flush them out for good.

Any therapy mentioned in the protocol may be of use. Counselling and letting go of any shame or guilt or negative beliefs about yourself are crucial.

Forgiveness plays a huge part. It can be hard but remember who you are doing this for; you.

If you hold onto grudges or judgement, you hold onto that abuser's energy. To hold something *against* them, means still linking to them, right?

Forgiveness is letting go and moving away from harm, and so you let them go and you forgive people, for you, not for them.

And it does not mean condoning what abusers did, it just means you are done suffering and you are claiming back your life and your bladder-space.

**You are flushing them out of your system.**

**A reminder of some energies linked to the bladder:**

- Frustration/Anger
- Irritation
- Fear/Terror/Worry/Anxiety
- Emotional blockages
- Desertion/Abandonment
- Pissed-offness
- Piss-takers/Abusers/Controllers/Narcissists/Taboo-Makers
- Sexual abuse/Rape/Not saying NO when you wanted to
- Being 'too nice'
- Inauthenticity
- Bed-wetting
- Bullying
- Piss-taking/Making a joke of you/Negative sarcasm
- Any emotional impact that shook you
- Self-loathing
- Disconnection to self and body
- Alcoholism
- Heavy smoking
- Poverty Belief
- Being a victim

In my metaphysical book, I delve much deeper but for now, you have the basic knowledge and tools to help your bladder be free.

Good luck. You got this.

Speak out safely and get professional help if needed.

**You are not alone.**

Remember that for any bladder pain, please, do seek medical help to identify any physical problems first. For emotional issues related to bladder frequency, do seek help from good therapists or reach out to someone you trust.

Metaphysics may be new to you, so adopt a few tools and increase from there. Your healing journey will improve greatly when dealt with at all levels.

## Tips to help clear blockages at all levels

### Physical

- Do a detox program (avoid damaging foods and drinks)
- Movement in the fresh air in nature
- Dry skin body brushing, salt baths and holistic treatments
- Swimming in cold water, ice baths, cold showers
- Deep sleep

### Emotional

Identify the feeling and blocked emotion you wish to clear. Naming it brings it up to the surface.

Rub your hands together and take a deep breath in. Hold your breath as you rub your lower back. Breathe out loudly as you wipe your hands off your spine to the ground. Have the intention to clear the emotion out. Do the same thing but this time rub a magnet clockwise on your belly with the intention of clearing the bladder.

## Mental

Identify the negative self-talk, phrases and belief patterns then say them out loud. Then state: this is not my truth and this program is now deleted.

Then counteract it with its opposite, so a power phrase for each negative phrase.

So if you identified:
I'm so pissed off that I get ill all the time!
Delete that and now reinforced with:

I'm grateful to be so vibrant.

Or

I'm so fat and ugly no wonder I can't find anyone!
to
My body is amazing and I love myself.

Repeat positive affirmations daily to train your thoughts to be helpful.

## Spiritual

Identify your deep-rooted beliefs. Decide if they are truly helpful and pulling you toward your best life or away from it. This includes letting go of traditions, religions, self-belief patterns and taboos that no longer suit you.

See your roots go deep into the earth and state:

I am part of nature and this is my home. I am present.

Do regular meditations.

**Aura**

To clear your energy field, stay away from things that depress you. Use sage to cleanse your space and your aura. Have salt baths. Have regular energy/holistic treatments. Smile. Laugh. Love.

A quick way to get answers from your body is to ask it. Until you get a great connection and just know the answers, here are a few ways to test.

- Body swaying. Stand straight, ask your body the question and see if you sway slightly forward then it is yes, a positive answer. If you lean slightly backwards then it is no, a negative answer.

- Muscle-testing. Someone else can muscle test you, so they would push gently down on your outstretched arm. Staying strong is a yes and if your arm gives way, it means no.

- Self-muscle-testing. There are several ways. Easiest is to form a circle by touching your thumb and forefinger together. Do it on each hand and link them up. If you can pull them apart easily it is a no, if they resist it is a yes.

- Use a pendulum that you dedicated to body communication. If it turns clockwise it means yes, anticlockwise means no.

Enjoy exploring ways to communicate with your body.

*Ah, good, I didn't wander off too far in my metaphysical realm.*

*And I brought you back safely.*

*Let's move on.*

## 12- Medical Protocol

Cystitis *is* a big deal.

It's wise to have your bladder checked medically if you have issues, especially recurring ones, to rule out any obvious bladder problems.

If you have cystitis or symptoms of cystitis, do go to the doctor and at least get a urine sample tested to check for bacteria. These aren't always accurate, but still worth doing and if it is confirmed that you have an infection, then do take antibiotics to help your body combat the germ.

If your doctor is unsympathetic or is of no help, then change your doctor.

If you are in a position to do so, get a camera in the bladder and be awake during the procedure so that you can see it for yourself. This will rule out several potential bladder issues.

Have an ultrasound of a full bladder and an empty bladder so they can check you are emptying properly and see the position of the bladder.

An MRI scan is also useful, as is one with a dye/contrast to track your waterworks, so fluid in the kidneys, tubes and bladder.

Antibiotics will only help to get rid of bacteria, not a virus, not candida, not a fallen bladder, not blockages or other major bladder malfunctions.

If you have recurring cystitis symptoms, even if nothing shows up in the urine, insist on being referred to a urologist, a so-called bladder expert.

If the specialist is arrogant and of no use, ask for a second opinion from another.

You are in charge of your body and your health, but the medical team does have an important part to play, especially in diagnosing bladder issues that they can test for such as cancer, fallen, neuro, leucoplakia, stones, or infections.

A sympathetic doctor and a useful urologist definitely form a part of our A-Team.

## 13- Posture Protocols

A good posture is important for so many reasons, physically and metaphysically. Standing tall, chest out, head up, empowers us, but hunched and looking down, victimises us.

When we stand in what I call a 'correct standing posture', one that humans are designed to be in, then all the organs sit in the right place and support each other. We are properly stacked.

If we lean forward too much or overly push out our hips, then our bladder and womb are not quite where they are supposed to be and gravity will tug at them.

Correct posture plays a part in keeping the bladder in place with the support it needs.

Sitting down posture is important too, for your back especially, and also your pelvis or any pelvic organs, including the bladder. We don't want to squash the bladder, so when sitting cross-legged or with legs outstretched, pull you bum cheeks apart slightly, pulling your flesh away from your sitting-bones, and tilt your pelvis forward and then back to find a comfortable neutral position.

The lying down position is important too although less as it gravity doesn't tug so much. I found the most comfortable is to lie on my front or side with a pillow under the knee/leg of the direction I'm facing. This seems to relieve pressure from the pelvic area.

*Explore and discover your favourite standing, sitting and lying position and write them in your journal.*

It's important to not stand or sit for too long, keep the blood and lymph flow active. And do move once you feel uncomfortable, as discomfort or pain is your body sending you signals to change something.

By now, you are more in tune with your body, so allow it to guide you to correct posture, and in the meantime, I recommend finding an experienced yoga or Pilates teacher and learn a few basic moves to improve your posture and your core muscle strength, and then practice them regularly.

The core muscles are the ones that look like a tight belt around your lower tummy and hips. They are deep inside and not bulky like muscles that you see, they are there to help keep the pelvis in shape and protect the organs and your spine. It tightens around that area to secure it, like a belt.

A strong core will definitely help bladder health. It will also help with good posture. It will help with all your body, as your main energy centre is in your lower belly, between the diaphragm and the sacral chakras.

In martial arts, we call this our powerhouse, or chi reserve.

When you exercise, it is important to keep your core muscles tight to hold your organs and spine in place. When you lift anything heavy, bend your knees, tighten your core and breathe out with the effort.

Ensure you have a strong core before doing heavy weight lifting or vigorous exercise. We want to avoid overusing your muscles or putting too much strain on your pelvic area. We need to slowly strengthen the core and all inner muscles, not over-exhaust them or push them too hard too soon and rip or weaken them.

I suggest you find a fitness instructor or a yoga teacher to show you how to strengthen your core muscles and body.

There are plenty of core strengthening exercises you can find online or in books so I won't be putting those here, as I still think it is best to be shown how to do these properly first by a professional.

**Warning:**

if you have a fallen bladder, do not jump up and down, run or do strenuous exercise. Get advice from a doctor or urologist you trust about exercise, even pelvic floor exercises. A good posture should help with avoiding getting this condition but check with your medical team if you have any grades of fallen bladder.

The Bladder A-Team has a strong core and awesome posture and is aware of the body at all times.

## 14- Exercise Protocols

We are designed to move.

There are countless reasons why exercise is crucial to us, but I will stick to the relevant reasons for bladder health, although we are all connected so movement is good for our body at all levels.

Because we are designed to move daily and walk a lot, some of our systems rely on movement. One of those is our lymph system; the drains. They are tubes and nodes, like junctions or stations that link the tubes together, and run all through our body.

This system has no pressure to help it along; the heart is a pump that pushes the blood, the lungs have a diaphragm that pushes the air, the bladder has muscles that push the urine, but our lymph was designed so that movement pushes that fluid along.

The fluid in the lymph is a carrier for gunk, germs, and anything we don't need anymore. They are garbage trucks picking up loose rubbish and disposing of it.

So, the lymph needs to be activated daily and exercise is the best way.

Movement, gravity, and shaking up, as well as deep massages and skin brushing, will help push the liquid along the lymph system and be sweated out.

- **Lymphatic System Protocol:**

  - Take deep breaths regularly as oxygen helps move the lymph along.

  - Drink plenty as hydration helps move the lymph along.

  - Avoid eating, drinking, inhaling, wearing or touching toxins in the first place.

  - Jump up and down for a minute each morning to shake the lymph along.

  - Do dry-skin brushing every day: use a natural body brush and massage your body upwards on dry skin. Start with the feet and brush upwards up your legs, hips, butt, tummy, back, boobs, then brush down your arms and neck towards your heart.
  The lymph will release its garbage through sweat glands and then

into the bloodstream for the liver and kidneys to deal with, so the more you sweat it out, the better for our bladder.

- Have cold showers. Cold helps to contract the muscles and the small veins and then the heat helps to open them up, this acts as a pumping action for the lymph. Start with a hot shower then go straight to cold, then back to hot, and then finish your shower with cold. Aim for 1 minute under the cold shower, or more if you can. Do this every morning. Swimming in cold water is also good for the lymph, but do ensure you dry and warm up fast afterwards, as our bladders don't like the cold or sitting in damp clothing.

- Have deep tissue or drainage massages; often if it hurts, that's usually good. I find a Thai Massage is good for the lymph system; I end up with bruises though, as it involves a lot of pressure on the blocked lymph nodes.

- **Exercising Protocols**

I don't believe in the recommended rules of how much exercise to do and when.

*Just move.*

When our bodies were designed, I'm sure it wasn't told we have to go to a gym and do 30 minutes of vigorous exercise five days a week. It was designed to move, a lot, and on a daily basis.

Moving could mean: walking at different paces depending on the reason; running; sprinting; climbing trees or rocks; cave exploring; swimming; lifting stuff; building things; stretching and bending to gather food;

fighting, in modern times we could practice martial arts or boxing; and, having sex.

If you like gyms, that's fine, but they are unnatural, indoors and full of air conditioning, so don't associate exercise with gyms, government recommendations or punishment. I go there only when I want to do specific lifting of weights, and I wear a scarf or a towel around my neck and nose to combat the cold air conditioning. Getting cold air blown on you whilst you are sweating is really not a great idea, especially if your throat or sinuses are a weak area.

See exercise as movement; a natural state for our body. Listen to your body and follow its advice, don't push yourself, and do protect yourself, this is how:

- Ensure you are clean before you exercise, we don't want anything on your knickers being pushed up your precious holes with the friction.

- Wear loose knickers and loose trousers/jogging pants, cotton, hemp or bamboo preferred.

- Breathe deeply and regularly, so don't hold your breath during movement.

- Drink plenty of water during and after exercise, not energy drinks or protein powders, just water, or water with good quality aloe vera or organic coconut water.

- Little and often is best, no need for hours at classes, in a gym, or running.

- If sitting at a desk or watching TV for too long, get up and jump up and down for 1 minute(hold your tummy as you do so), or do a few yoga positions, or stretches, that's enough; just get moving.

- After exercising, if you sweat, then shower and change into fresh knickers and clothes, don't sit in damp sweaty clothes. If you can't shower, then at least do the flannel-lick and put on fresh knickers. If you don't have fresh knickers, then you can use an organic cotton sanitary towel to ensure the damp gusset doesn't touch your precious holes.

- After exercising and whilst you are still warm, do some deep stretching: hold each stretch for 1 minute, as it takes about that time for the lymph to flush out the acid build-up that the exercise created.
The acid build-up is what causes those cramps and painful post-exercise muscles. So, stretching will help clear out the toxins, as will drinking plenty of water.

- Eat some high-quality protein after exercise to help your muscles repair, obviously not dairy. When we do strenuous exercise or weights, we tear our muscle fibres, and they rebuild bigger and stronger; the building blocks are amino acids, proteins and water. Ensure good nutrition and hydration after vigorous or bodybuilding exercise.

## 15- Environmental Protocols

This crosses over with other protocols but worth mentioning on its own.

Who you spend your time with socially will be classed as community protocol.

*This is more how you move within your world.*

**Weather**

Be mindful of the weather that day or if you go abroad in a different environment than you are used to. Take precautions. If it is hot then use appropriate sun-cream, wear a hat, seek shade and drink more water.

If it is cold or damp, ensure to keep warm and bring umbrellas or waterproof outer clothing, and if you do get wet, do change into dry underwear and clothing as soon as possible so not to sit in a damp gusset!

If it is icy or treacherous use tools to help you such as walking sticks, special shoe attachments or snow-chains on your car.

Avoid walking barefoot on cold tiles, as this can cause irritation to the bladder.

**So be aware of how you can damage your spine and bladder and how to take measures to lessen the chances of you damaging yourself.**

**Avoid Falls/Impact/Potential Risks**

If you are of heavier weight or have bladder or womb issues of any kind I would suggest not going down any water slides, the impact of the water shooting up the precious holes at such allure can be problematic. You could also damage your coccyx, lower back and nerves endings, linked to possible bladder issues.

If you are walking in damp, wet or icy conditions, ensure proper footwear and use Nordic walking poles or a walking stick to help balance yourself, and be well-grounded and sure-footed, as any fall could impact your spine and bladder area.

Before walking down any stairs, take a moment to pull in your tummy muscles and pull up your spine and hold onto a ramp if possible.

Be aware of the potential dangers without being scared of becoming a victim to them.

If you are taking part in potentially dangerous activities, truly think if you want to and if it is worth the risk of falling or damaging yourself.

Potential dangers could be any fairground ride, jerky rollercoasters, slides, horse-riding, rollerblading, roller-skating, ice-skating, contact sports, jumping or diving in water from a height, riding a bike if you are not used to it, walking down stairs with long skirt or trousers that could trip you up, or even perching on a pointy surface.

If your environment isn't safe or could be problematic, leave. So, for example, walk away if a fight breaks out, or if you are somewhere that makes you uncomfortable.

If someone or something is frustrating and angering you, get away or take precautions. Especially if you are subjected to situations or people that annoy you chronically, then in order to avoid metaphysical cystitis, do take countermeasures. You can think of what those may be depending on the situation. For example, getting good earplugs if your partner snores or you have noisy neighbours.

And have difficult conversations when they will help clear the air.

Be aware of all that's going on in your environment and social life so that you can make the best decisions about your health and keeping your bladder happy.

**Note**: this is the newest protocol that I created as a result of going down a huge water-slide on holiday with my family and I was teased for not wanting to do it. My cousin said 'well what the worst that can happen? Just do it' And so I did but I should have listened to my intuition.

So what happened was that I broke my coccyx that led to months of urology issues.

The worst that could have happened is dying, as not long after that I read that a couple went down a similar water-slide but face first and the force broke the man's neck and he died on the spot.

The woman was hurt but didn't die, but had to then deal with losing her husband.

So I'm not being a kill-joy or pissing on your bomb-fire here, but just be aware of your environment and listen to your intuition, never mind about the teasing or goading. Listen to your inner voice as maybe it knows best.

## 16- Community Protocols

Who you spend your time with *will* affect your health and quality of life.

Your environment and social life matters.

There is a saying '**monkey see, monkey do**'.
Some new monkeys were introduced into the wild and they survived by observing the local monkeys and copied them.
So surround yourself with happy healthy monkeys.

Avoid regular contact with people who drink too much, smoke, have no clue or desire to know about health or personal development, have no sympathy or understanding of women's issues, who are bullies and make you feel small; you get the idea.

It is said that if you want to be rich, hang out with much richer people than you and study their habits, copy them and the more you bask in their frequencies, the quicker your own antenna will morph to adopt a similar range and attract more money.

The same is true with health. It is much easier to make healthy food choices and not smoke or get pissed (getting pissed, slang for drinking too much alcohol, another linguistic clue that the bladder doesn't like it) if you are surrounded by those who also avoid it, or who don't influence you to do it.

There is no need to have to say no to cigarettes when none of your friends smoke.

However, continuously surround yourself with people who drink, smoke and have no respect for their health, and you will be consistently fighting against it or give in and lower your own frequencies to fit in.

**I'm hoping seeing as you are still with me on this book journey, that you now understand the importance of putting your health first because, without good health, we cannot pursue our dreams or experience the vibrant life that we crave.**

Evaluate your buddies and social circles and walk away from the toxic ones.

Find new buddies. Harsh? Maybe, but in my opinion, it's crucial.

In an ideal world, you will influence those friends to join you in a healthy regime, and change the world one person at a time, starting with you.

The way to enlighten the world is to be the lightest in it, and then others will gravitate toward you also wanting that light, that health, and copy you.

You will become the healthy monkey that others will observe and mimic.

Remember these protocols are to bring your full A-Game to your life and community. It doesn't mean you have to make all the changes and not all at once, it can be a gradual painless process.

I'm not saying to ditch all your friends that no longer suit you right now, but start being OK with distancing yourself and look for fresher communities, surrounding yourself with like-minded people.

It's OK too to still have the occasional night out with people who are toxic, enjoy it but be mindful.

And I'm not saying you can never get pissed or have a fag (UK slang for cigarette as I believe it may mean something quite different in the US!) or unprotected sex, I'm saying be mindful and understand what it takes for 100% bladder health, and then decide how you are going to adapt your lifestyle and how many of the A-Team checkboxes you are prepared to tick on a regular basis at this stage in your life.

You don't need to make 100% changes to get results. Any percentage of change is welcome and can provide a basis for a further increase later.

*What could just 5% changes make in your bladder health?*
*Write this sentence stem in your journal and have a ponder:*

**With just 5% extra health, I would…**

You may not be ready at all, or even agree with some protocols, and that is OK, but leave an open mind. Maybe one day you will be ready or want to read it again and implement more of the changes.

For now, we are learning all the protocols, to familiarise them.

I suggest that you implement some of them now.

If you want full life-changing effects now, then apply them all and stick to them.

## Welcome To Our Jungle

By buying this book, you are now part of our *happy bladder* community. You now have instant access to a thriving group of people from across the globe that have read this book and embarked on improving their bladder health.

I have created a closed Facebook group for people on happy bladder journeys, and you are now invited.

Welcome to the jungle of happy-bladder monkeys.

To access it, you will need a Facebook account (free) and you will need to apply to join the group (also free, press the button 'join group'), the administrators will then permit you as part of the tribe.

Once in this community, you can liaise with others, discuss the book, any challenges, ask or offer help, ask for support, share tips and things that are working, and even meet up and make new friends.

The Facebook group name is called:
**The Happy Bladder Tribe**

It is important to get advice from those who have conquered their nemesis and to have a safe place to discuss all things related to bladder health without judgement or taboos. It is important to talk to people who understand.

No more hiding away embarrassed or not talking about cystitis or other women's issues because they may be related to private parts, toilets, sex, menstruation, rape, hormones, shame/guilt, painful memories, and other subjects we have been trained not to discuss or to keep private, well not anymore.

Taboos are restrictions and not health-promoting.

**With this book, we smash taboos and render them irrelevant.**

You do not need to suffer in silence, you don't need to suffer at all, and you don't need to hold onto anything anymore.

We hear you, we see you, and we understand.

Come to the community and tell us your bladder story. Share what is working or has worked for you, because that one person is waiting to read that.

The idea of building the A-Team is to understand everything that causes bladder issues and why and then counteract those. You don't have to do all these all the time. You have to live your life, this is about freedom, not more restrictions, but it is about making choices to increase bladder health and not deplete it.

As long as you know that you are engaging in trigger issues and going against the bladder, that is already a massive step; knowledge is key. Then comes the application, so take countermeasures to balance out the negative impact.

For example, on your date night, enjoy that romantic meal eating all you want, having too much alcohol, a sneaky cigarette or a full-on snog with someone who has been drinking and smoking, and that's the spice of life, enjoy it, but do be aware that is four ticks in the trigger boxes, so counteract it by ensuring you tick plenty in the A-Team too, and be mindful of your fulcrum.

So, when you get back to the hotel or bedroom with this date and you decide it's sexy time, then engage in the sexual hygiene protocol as much as possible and drink plenty of water. Have some aloe vera before bed to negate the effects of the meal. And please, don't wear a thong on that date! Commando is fine, or big comfy cotton knickers and then go to the toilet before sex and ditch them.

I have devised, later in this book, an easy to read checklist for boxes in the trigger team and boxes in the A-Team, to make it easier to recollect.

## And…breathe.

*I know it's a lot to take in. Well done, we made it through a big chapter.*

Remember, you don't need to make all these changes now, you don't have to follow each protocol exactly. You can pick and choose, or do them all.

If you apply every protocol and sub-protocol on a daily basis, you will absolutely change your life: it can't be any other way.

You can still change your bladder health by applying just a few. If you are overwhelmed and only want a few changes, for now, I have devised a quick way.

Identify which type of cystitis you suffer from regularly and apply the protocols that will help the most.

**Bacterial, viral infection or sexual cystitis**
Toilet protocol
Sexual protocol
Daily hygiene protocol
Hydration protocol

**Candida, IBS, overactive/oversensitive cystitis**
Nutrition protocol
Hydration protocol
Toilet protocol

**Metaphysical cystitis**
Metaphysical Protocol
Hydration Protocol

**Medically induced cystitis, diabetes-related, pregnancy or abnormal pressure, fallen bladder, bladder cancer, bladder stones**
Medical protocol
Posture Protocol
Hydration Protocol

**Note**: all types of bladder issues will be helped by all the protocols, so do ensure you familiarise yourself with this entire chapter.

Make notes in your journal, put bullet points on your wall, do whatever it takes to get this information drummed in.

Start making changes now. The more protocols you follow, the quicker your journey to happy bladder health will be.

**The A-Team employs all the protocols, now.**

## Chapter 6 Keynotes

- There are 16 major protocols with further sub-protocols for **building your Bladder A-Team**

- **Knowledge is key**. We can no longer sweep sensitive stuff under the carpet, or turn a blind eye to things that will affect our health.

- Dairy and artificial sweeteners are *seriously* detrimental to our health.

- Any abuse suffered by animals, the environment, or people making your products, clothing, food and drink will affect us too.

- Energy begets similar energy. You are what you buy, eat, drink, inhale, touch, and associate with.

- We vote with our money, what are you condoning?

- Our bladders are affected by our lives at all levels: physical, posture, nutritional, mental, sexual, emotional, spiritual, social, and environmental.

- Smashing taboos, talking about the unspeakable and clearing out dark secrets, will make space in our energetic bladder.

- It's my (the author's) job to inform you of all issues that could affect bladders, no matter how controversial, non-conventional, or if it pushes your buttons. It is your job (the reader) to be open-minded and to implement the protocols. We are a team.

## Action! Interactive bit, it's your turn:

1. What have you read in this chapter that really made you think?

2. Were you aware of how detrimental dairy was?

3. What nutritional changes are you prepared to make now? In the future?

4. In your journal, list which items from each of the 16 major protocol sections that you are going to do from now on.

5. Write down in your journal any strong feelings or memories that reading this chapter brought up for you.

6. Evaluate the people you spend most of your time with and rate their toxicity levels.

7. Do you spend time with toxic books, computer games, magazines, media, TV channels, social media, people, too much bad inner talk? How can you improve the quality of your time and activities?

8. Join our Private Facebook Group and introduce yourself.

9. Ensure to access the *Products & Services Reference*, to know what products, cooking utensils, food, drink and clothing I use and where to source them.

So, now we have explored the protocols, we know how to build your Bladder A-Team.

We know that living cystitis-free is possible and you now have all the tools you need.

You are comfortable and rocking the driver's seat!

Exciting, right? Let this chapter *really* sink in and make more notes in your journal.

* * *

OK, notes done so let's just congratulate ourselves on the knowledge we have gained so far. Awesome job!

*Phew! That was the longest stretch of our journey, so well done. I'm glad we shared the driving!*

Let's have a cup of herbal tea and a stretch and then meander onto the next chapter…

Ready?

OK, let's mozzie on down to communicating with your bladder.

# CHAPTER 7

# Setting Up Proper Bladder Communication

It's time to get in touch with your body and listen to signs.

You and your body are a team: reconnect.

**The better the connection, the better the flow.**

When we are in chronic pain, especially frustrating cystitis, we tend to disconnect from our body. This is a common reaction. We train ourselves to leave our body as it is too painful, scary or shaming to be present in it during agony or abuse.

Fear also plays a part in wanting to leave our body.

We say that that we *shit* ourselves, or *shat* ourselves when we mean we got so scared. So fear very much lives in the intestines as well as in the bladder

This is particularly true in rape or sexual abuse of any kind, which has an energy link to the bladder. Abuse also has links to the womb and the bowels.

Whilst this coping mechanism is useful to deal immediately with nasty experiences, it does have long term implications. With cystitis, it means we ignore our bladder.

We haven't been fully present in our body for years, probably since our first cystitis bout. This disconnects us and we no longer communicate easily, resulting in full-blown cystitis, which may have been dealt with a lot earlier if we knew it was coming.

How can you love your bladder and really listen, if you are not fully connected to it?

If the pain goes on for the long term and disconnecting happens often, you could end up hating your body. Your mind-body-spirit connection is severed, or at least, wobbled. Fighting against the body, living in anger, frustration and pissed-off-ness will create a vicious cycle, and more of that frequency will be applied to the bladder.

Think of your bladder or recurring cystitis as a child, wanting your attention, or your beloved pet clawing at you for a pick-up, what would you say to that child or pet? Would you scream, telling them you can't stand them, that it's not fair, and why are they plaguing your life, then ignore them and leave them? Probably not, so from now on, let's not do that to our body either.

It's time to view and treat your body the way you would your best friend, and your health will benefit greatly.

### The Importance of Self-Love

Self-love is crucial to health and creating a fulfilling life. There are many paths back to self-love.

I say *back*, as usually we are born with it and it gets beaten out of us by society and expectations.

I have created a meditation to help you and doing it regularly will help strengthen the bond back to yourself. Following all the protocols will also encourage self-love.

**Repeat these statements:**

I AM SAFE

I AM BLISS

I AM CALM

I AM LOVE

MY BLADDER IS HAPPY

I LOVE MY BLADDER

I FORGIVE MYSELF

ALL IS WELL

I AM PRESENT

I AM SELF-LOVE

* * *

## The Importance of Forgiveness

Forgiveness is crucial. We hold onto too many grudges, negative stories, and thoughts of revenge, and it's time to let those go. Releasing shackles of blame and vengeance will free us.

The most important person to forgive is yourself, for everything. Every decision you made has resulted in the person you are today, and you are amazing.

It's time to get to know and accept that amazing-ness again.

Forgiving other people is also important, not for their sake but for yours. Again, the clue is in the language, if you hold something against someone, a grudge, you need to be close enough to hold that something against them; you have to be in their energy field, using up so much of your own precious energy to keep it there.

Energetically, for you to keep the grudge against their energy-field is self-draining, and it doesn't harm them, it hurts you, and your loved ones watching you suffer.

Only you can release that energy link, forgiving them is key; again, a clue in the language, to forgive is to give it away (it is *for* giving).

By forgiving them, you severe the energetic link and give back what is theirs and you keep what is yours, and you are free to move on.

Forgiveness does not mean condoning their actions or making them right, it just means you walk away because you are more important.

Your health is more important than any grudge or hunger for revenge.

Life is precious, live it in your own space, for you, and find that self-love.

It starts by releasing all the energies that are not yours. Then by recalling lost or forgotten parts of you including those are left out in the cold, because revenge is cold, another clue in language; best served cold.

It is not OK that people hurt you, but wanting revenge or relentlessly thinking about it, will only fill you with negative energy and attract more of that energy to you.

Trust me, I know; if you can't forgive that bully from school, you will attract more bullies as an adult. Energy begets similar energy. What energy lives in you?

*Let it go* (permission to sing is granted).

Fill your whole body with self-love and feel your life change.

There are many ways to increase your self-love. Over the years I found several and I love using mirrors, it has a way to get a deeper connection. I first found mirror work when I was doing a sacred geometry course, and have come across many practitioners who encourage mirror work since.

## Look In The Mirror

One way to start forgiving and reconnecting to yourself is by looking in the mirror:

It doesn't take much time and can be super effective.

Look in the mirror into your eyes, study them, and then study your face, your body.

Look into your eyes and state the following, and fill in the blanks, anything will do, it can be the same phrases or different ones.

You can stop at three or go on for as many as you want. Do this every morning for at least 2 weeks, or however long until you feel a positive change. If you are in public, you can say it in your head and imagine looking at your eyes.

I forgive myself for_____

I forgive myself for _____

I forgive myself for _____

**Examples related to bladder health:**

I forgive myself for eating inflammatory foods too often.

I forgive myself for ignoring the signs that cystitis was coming.

I forgive myself for not speaking out when I was abused.

I forgive myself for staying too long with a partner who did not respect me.

I forgive myself for being pissed off at myself.

I forgive myself for all the times I left my body.

I forgive myself for how badly I talk to myself.

I forgive myself for having been bullied.

I forgive myself for the abuse I have put my body through.

I forgive myself for my ignorance and lack of self-respect.

I forgive myself for saying *yes* when I wanted to say *no*.

I forgive myself for holding things and grudges against others or myself.

I forgive myself for drinking and smoking too much.

I forgive myself for the times I was too shy to go to the toilet.

I forgive myself for using fake cystitis as an excuse to get out of something.

**And end with this phrase:**

I forgive myself for *everything,* as every decision and action I made led to the person I am today, and I love the person I am now.

Now, applaud yourself, remember your amazingness, gaze into your eyes and again, fill in the blanks:

I am amazing because _____
I am amazing because _____
I am amazing because_____

**Examples for bladder health:**

I am amazing for taking these steps to self-love.

I am amazing for applying these protocols.

I am amazing for putting myself first, at last.

I am amazing because even through all the pain, I have not given up hope.

I am amazing because I'm aligning myself with my true path.

I am amazing because I have forgiven everything.

I am amazing because I love myself.

I am amazing because I have strong boundaries.

I am amazing because I no longer allow anyone to abuse me.

I am amazing because I have the power to say no.

I am amazing because I love my bladder.

I am amazing just for being me.

And finally, commit to yourself, make a promise: look deeply into your eyes and make this true.

I promise that _____
I promise that _____
I promise that _____

**Bladder health examples:**

I promise that I will do this mirror connection every day.

I promise that I will follow these protocols.

I promise that I will actively work on my self-love.

I promise that I will love my bladder.

I promise that I come first and that's OK.

I promise that no one will bully me ever again.

I promise to be more present in my body, and in my life.

I promise that I will align myself with optimal happiness.

I promise to drink at least 2 litres of clean water every day.

I promise to eat the right foods every day.

\* \* \*

## The Importance of Presence

When you are in self-love, you listen more, your senses are more active, you feel more nurtured, more grounded, more real and safer. You have more energy, more excitement, and you get your 'joie de vivre', your mojo back.

Remember a time when you were with someone having a conversation, you had something important to say and you were devoted to this connection, but that person started looking around, distracted, or paying attention to another girl across the room, or worse, looking at their phone, or even walking away.

*How did you feel?*

That person was not present, they may have been physically there with you, but their energy was not.

Now, imagine you are having this conversation again, but this time the person is fully facing you, maybe holding your hand, looking directly at you. No phones or wandering eyes, they smile and nod as you talk, they get closer to you as you connect.

*How does that feel?*

This person is totally present with you, in body, mind, and energy.

That is how you want to treat yourself, to be there for you like that.

To be there for others like that.

Practice being present with whoever you converse with, even the bus driver as you get your ticket or the person at the checkout in the supermarket, smile, look at them, really acknowledge them, and respect the space you are currently sharing.

Humans crave true connection and ironically in this modern world where virtual communication and internet-relationships are so rife, where it is easier to connect with people globally online than ever, we are losing our touch-connection, our actual presence.

Don't be that person who looks around, distracted by so many things, be the one who looks at the other person and offers them presence.

Our bladder is no different because every cell that makes up our body is connected, at every level, not just the physical. Energies bond to similar frequencies, so if you direct hate or anger to any part of yourself, *all* the cells will get that message and react in kind.

If you say to yourself that you are ugly or you are ill, eventually you will be ugly and ill because your body is designed to obey your principal thoughts and loudest commands.

Your thoughts create things. Your energy dictates the quality of your cells. You can think yourself ill and you can think yourself healthy, so be mindful of your thoughts, your beliefs, and your mental activity. One way to do that is to be fully present in your body and observe everything.

You are the director of your movie, of your life. Is it going to be a horror, a comedy, or a feel-good film?

It is time to come home to your body. You want to listen to your bladder the way you would like to be listened to.

It is now time to turn your nemesis into your best friend, deal with your problems together.

**An example of when I was not present properly:**

I studied cystitis and the bladder for decades and understood the theory, but sometimes I didn't pay enough attention to my findings and did things anyway. I went against protocols because you know, I'm (partly) human, resulting in cystitis.

*Then I truly understood as I experienced the theory, solidifying the lesson.*

When I lived in London, my new boyfriend came over. We went to bed, to sleep only, as it takes me a while to agree to sex with new partners. I was having a period and too embarrassed to tell him, and I still had issues going to the toilet if someone else was there. So, I stayed the night with a dirty tampon (that was the last time I ever used one), and I held on to my pee until he left the next morning.

By the time I went to the loo, I had bacterial cystitis and had to go to the doctors for antibiotics. I knew in theory that period hygiene and not holding onto pee were crucial in bladder health, but I hadn't experienced it yet.

I then worked on my issues with toilet or menstruation embarrassment. I ensured that wherever I was, or whomever I was with, I would go to the loo, and take my time and ensure period and toilet hygiene protocol every time. That was the last time I got cystitis due to poor period hygiene or holding on too long before peeing.

Another lesson well-learned was having sex with a new boyfriend (years later) for the first time and not being brave enough to say I wanted us to shower first, and we needed to, as we had been out all night partying. The next day I was itchy and got sexual and bacterial cystitis.

That was the last time I had cystitis through poor sexual hygiene and not speaking out. I did work on myself to ensure that I put my health first and have those awkward conversations.

Years later I did get sexual cystitis that led to bacterial due to lack of poor sexual hygiene, but not because I was too embarrassed to have the talk but because I got too drunk to look after myself properly or ensure sexual protocols or to push him away.

That is the last time I get cystitis or become vulnerable due to alcohol. I learned a really valuable lesson that night that helped me on my journey of self-forgiveness and self-love. I'm now very aware of the energy a man leaves behind and because, *finally,* I love myself enough to put me first, and also because I'm done attracting selfish Beep-heads as lovers. There is a great pagan saying: 'when in doubt, leave it out.'

When I love and respect myself to a high degree that is when I will be attracted to men who are deserving of my love and who respect me too.

**I have a feeling that we can only let in people to love us at the same level we love ourselves. Hence self-love is crucial.**

I'm sharing these stories in the hope they will impact you at a deeper level, so that the theory is enough for you to really apply these protocols, and you don't have to suffer cystitis through ignorance or embarrassment.

During my long journey, I did have signals, 'mini-cystitis', and counteracted them immediately. You have suffered for decades probably with a weakened bladder so it will take some time to learn how to treat it well, and that is OK. You got this.

If you find a new trigger for cystitis, do share it with us in the Facebook private group, because sharing is caring. Also by writing down and voicing your findings, it helps that information to truly sink deeper for you too, so it is a win-win situation and I like those.

Your bladder is not a victim and neither are you. It is time to stand up for yourself and speak out. If a partner is not prepared to shower or do their bit to help your bladder health, then they have no right touching you.

R.E.S.P.E.C.T. for yourself, and command it from others. This is where social decluttering comes into its own.

Ditch the shit.

**Ditch *all* douche-bags.**

Douches are no good for our bits and no good as boyfriends.

* * *

## The Importance of Being Earnest

Earnest means showing a sincere and intense conviction.

I relate it here to being authentic (truthful, acting and behaving like the real you) and beyond that is being earnest. So, showing up in your life as your true self with sincere and intense conviction.

A conviction so strong that no one can shake you or morph you into their expectation.

A belief in yourself so unshakable that you can remain standing among any outside chaos, and not allow others' opinions, taboos or social expectations to throw you off your bladder-health course.

A conviction that you will put your health first and no longer put up with behaviours that lead you away from it and who you truly are.

## I see that as being totally unabashed.

As problems with honesty, authenticity and sincerity all have links to the bladder energetically, it is important to ensure you are true to yourself and others.

Your bladder no longer wants any inauthentic energies buried within it.

## Signals from the Bladder

So, let's go deeper into signs from your bladder that something is wrong before it's too late.

Depending on your preferred senses, there will be different systems to flag this up.

I have created a few here to give you ideas. Use these or invent your own that works for you. The idea is to build stronger communication between you and your bladder.

**Visual:** a flag system. See yourself as a lifeguard on your white wooden tower on a beautiful beach overlooking the calm blue ocean.

You have a pole in front of you with a flag on top. Green means all is well, orange means there is a problem coming, and red depicts danger. Your subconscious to conscious relay person is the lifeguard, the flag is the signal (what your bladder wants you to know), and the sea is the bladder (your waterworks).

What you want is a green flag, so blissful, happy. The sea ebbs and flows quietly, a few white birds flying over the horizon, the water is clear and all is well.

The orange flag is put up when the sea becomes rougher, noisier, and murkier, with a few large crashing waves and some debris. This means that cystitis is coming, or there is something bothering your waterworks, but there is still time to calm it before a full-on storm.

So the orange flag goes up, the lifeguard signals your consciousness and you tune in and work out what is going wrong and how to fix it, you agree to appease the waterworks. It's your bladder saying 'Hey! Help me, please!'

The red flag means danger. Either you have ignored the orange flag, or you did too much in one go, bypassing the orange straight to red alert. At this stage, the ocean is angry, dark, a tsunami devastating the beach, the lifeguard hanging onto a floating piece of his white tower, now torn to shreds by the typhoon that already hit, debris everywhere, vultures circling, threatening skies, horrific noise, the storm has done its damage and is still rampaging. This means you have full-blown cystitis or worse.

When you see the red flag, it is high time to deploy the *Bladder Rescue Team* and keep the faith, have hope, the storm will pass, and you will be able to clear up after it and return to a green flag beach, but for now you have to ride the storm, no choice.

This may sound silly if you haven't done visualisation or imagery work before, but trust me, it is a fantastic way of keeping in touch with your body and how your bladder is really doing.

**Aural:** if you are more into listening, then perhaps you would prefer sounds to images. Find an alarm in your head or on your phone that you can assign to your bladder. You want three sounds:

1. a soothing calm noise for the 'All is Well' signal.

2. a louder alarming sound as a warning bell that something is amiss, an 'SOS' call.

3. a loud, crashing alarm calling out the 'Mayday' signalling the storm has hit and the emergency rescue operation is urgent.

It could be simple as a triangle ding for sound 1, cymbals crashing for sound 2, and a full-on drumbeat for emergency sound 3, or more complicated, like an actual alarm sound or a designated song for each level.

You decide, play around, see what sounds right.

**Touch:** if you are more of a touchy-feely person, something simple will work like put your hands on your tummy above your bladder and feel changes in temperatures, sensations, tingling, pulsing.

Ask your bladder to show you how it feels on your hands when it is happy, sad, or angry. Tune in anytime by placing your hands over your bladder area and ask the question, 'bladder how are you feeling?', and pay attention to your hands.

You can even instruct your bladder what the signs are; bladder, if all is well, send a cooling sensation on my hands; if you need SOS, make it a tingling sensation, if you need emergency help, make my hands hot.

**Metas:** so for those of you already practising metaphysics, you may wish to pick something that resonates more with you. For example, buy a pendulum that you dedicate solely for communicating with your bladder. A good crystal for the bladder would be blue, for water, or orange or red relating to the local chakras.

I like Carnelian as that represents joy, so a happy bladder, but any crystal or any pendulum would be fine, as long as you choose it for your bladder.

Ask the pendulum clear questions: is my bladder happy? Yes or No. If yes, then all is well. If no, then ask why. Is it something I drank, ate, and then list the protocols until a 'yes' comes. Did I break the sexual hygiene protocol? Yes or no. And if it circles yes quite profoundly, take that as an emergency, and a rescue team is needed.

Another way would be to pick a special oracle deck of cards that you dedicate to your bladder (or womb) communication. It could be a water theme, so ocean or mermaids. Pick a card and read it to understand your bladder message, is it a 'calm card', or is it a 'help me now' card?

At some point with practice, you will naturally be reconnected to your body and then you will just know without the use of any tools. This is claircognizance. Until then, or even just for fun, do use a specific method to connect to your bladder.

Self-claircognizance feels amazing. This is where your body and you are one; an awesome team and experiencing life through self-love, self-respect, and presence.

See the meditation section for extra help.

**So, as a reminder, here are possible signals that the bladder is unhappy:**

- Headache
- Dehydration/Thirsty
- Stress

- Being angry or frustrated
- Worrying about money at a deep or chronic level (poverty belief)
- Acute or slight burning when you pee
- Involuntary squeeze/Spasm after peeing
- Bladder pain
- Discomfort in your lower body
- Electricity shooting up the urethra
- Being too cold
- Have cold or sore kidneys like punched in the lower back. If your kidneys are unhappy so may your bladder as it is the downfall and stored what the kidneys make.
- Blood in the urine
- Bloating, especially after eating certain trigger foods
- Irritability/Frustration/Anger
- Fever
- Being run down
- Itchy or sore vulva
- Thrush or trauma in the vagina
- Post-sex discomfort
- Knowing you have been exposed to germs, a feeling something isn't right
- Cramps
- Dark or smelly urine (unless you have eaten **asparagus** as this make your pee stink, but that is normal and should go away within approx. 24 hours)
- Needing to go frequently to the loo
- Not having much wee even though you feel you can't leave the toilet
- Doubled up with abdominal pain
- Fainting

- Shortness of breath
- Disconnection, feeling abandoned or lost
- Rat-Race, loss of control, if you feel you are living someone's else's life or fulfilling someone else's dreams, or in the wrong job, or with the wrong partner, or doing something simply because it is expected of you, if you are not in control of your life, then you are not totally in control of your health.
- Pissed-off, or being surrounded by piss-takers
- Calm demeanour, a mask to the world but underneath you are going crazy, not showing up in the world as the real you
- Lack of authenticity at any level

- **The swan effect**: my great-grandma Mémé Lili suffered from cystitis all her life. I was unable to help her as I didn't know then what I know now, but when I had it and she was around, she would give me a hot water bottle and say 'I understand, you must get it from me.' Cystitis is not genetically transferred, but metaphysically inherited family belief patterns can play a part.

Mémé Lili was a swan because she was so graceful and always doing things for others, never stopping for herself or looking after herself properly. So, to the outside, she looked graceful, swimming along, but underneath the water, her legs and feet were peddling fast to keep her afloat.

Looking back at her life, it is easy to see why she would have metaphysical and circumstantial cystitis.

Her mum died when she was 10, and her father sent her to a farmhouse to be in service, in the next village miles away up a mountain. Her wages were sent to her father, she never got any of it. She would sleep in the barn with the pigs, and work in the farmyard and then in the large farmhouse in service, in the kitchens, waiting the family table, housework. Her life was not her own at all. She learnt that she didn't matter and that life was just like that, you serve others, no matter what.

The only day she had off was Christmas day, where she was allowed to walk home, alone in the snow, to see her family, not that she really wanted to as her step-mother was wicked and the only thing she got for Christmas was an orange, for which she was grateful, then she walked back that night ready for work the next morning.

She was in service since her childhood, from 10 to 21 years old, as you were not an adult until then, and so had to obey your parents, guardians or employers.

Children, unless they were from well-off families, like the one she served, were expected to earn their keep. Sadly back then if the master of the house or his teenage sons wanted to touch you, there was no one to help you; you were considered their property. She didn't matter, she had no voice. Who knows the abuse she was probably subjected to; sexual, labour, verbal, and the levels of hygiene from sleeping in a barn and not having bath privileges.

When I asked her about her childhood or teenage years she would clam up and tears would fill her eyes. She just used to whisper that they were miserable times, and we don't talk about that. I found out basic facts from my Nan, her daughter.

Mémé Lili died at 92, her bladder and her body harboured so many dark, abusive secrets, for over 80 years, so it's no wonder that she suffered frequently with cystitis, even as an adult.

So if you are able to, do air out any nasty memories lurking within. She always gave to others, putting everyone else first gracefully, but always running around for other people, never believing that she could come first, not even in her own life.

If you feel like you are in service or in sacrifice to others the whole time, if you feel you are put upon, that is not a good place to be for your bladder health.

I learnt a lot from Mémé Lili, she was amazing. She taught me how to cook, how to garden, what herbs or mushrooms to gather, but her main lesson was about being graceful. She once said to me when I was huffing about something,

'Jenny, if you decide you are going to do something, do it with grace'.

I like that. The clue there is if *you decide* to do something, then gracefully and presently is the way, but if someone else is making you do something that isn't right, then sod grace and stand up for yourself.

We live in a world now of abundant health services, counselling, and protection, so do use them if needed.

Smile if you mean it, but don't fake it, fix the separation within first.

Be authentic, this will help your bladder.

Looking for joy outside of yourself, so feeling you need someone else, or have the perfect job to be happy, to fulfil or complete you, is counterproductive to the bladder, and so many other things.

In true self-love and presence, you are full and complete and can enjoy the company of others but do not rely on them for your own happiness and well-being.

**Self-love is not a woo-woo concept: it is crucial.**

Just to be clear, self-love does not mean selfish, or totally self-centred, that is classed as egocentric or narcissism.

True self-love means self-full and loving yourself in a healthy way that enhances your love frequency and presence, hence helping to light up the world.

Think of Mary Poppins, what a great example. She is proud, has great posture, and she gives no apology or explanation for who she is, she owns it. She helps others but not at her own cost, she knows exactly who she is and her worth. She has infinite value and owns that, and does not need validation or approval from anybody else, including her bosses.

She commands respect and exudes self-esteem, and I can't help but love her.

She also invented the best word ever, as a linguist I love that. OK, I know Mary Poppins is fictional (by Disney), but she exists at some level, and that's good enough for me.

So when you find yourself in a pickle just say:

'supercalifragilisticexpialidocious',

and that word will make you smile and stand up straight. And just doing that will do wonders for your quality of life. Good posture allows better flow and connection from the sun to the earth within us, as conduits of energy.

Smiling releases happy endorphins and infectious in a great way, sharing the love and connection.

Good posture also helps bladder health. So, there is a tiny link to Mary Poppins and bladder health. I did warn you even if the information is minutely relevant, it has a place in this book.

Being present happens when you are truly connected to your body, are habitually aware of all of your senses, and knowing who you are, where you are, and how you fit into this world authentically.

We all experience moments of presence, but then we miss-align and go off track.

**Presence is trainable.**

The great news is that higher frequencies vibrate faster and therefore influence the lower ones. So, that means if you can be fully present every day, even just for a moment, it will have a huge impact and will help you anchor it, so that you can access presence more often, until, one day in utopia, we all live from a present state, when this happens, there will be no wars, no abuse.

When totally present and in self-love, it is impossible to hurt another being, including animals or trees, because you understand that how you treat others is a reflection of how you treat yourself.

What value you give to others, reflects the amount of self-value that you harbour.

You understand that even though we are all unique and have our own lives and experiences to lead, we are still all made from the same source-energy and are all connected, and so harming others means harming yourself.

It feels awesome to experience true love, bliss and presence. Yes, agreed, what an idealist I am, and yes it could take a long time to reach that globally, but all that matters is your life, how you live, how high you can get your personal frequency to resonate, and how you choose to live your life, that's it.

The world gets changed one person at a time.

When you are present you can be centred even in chaos. Knowing that you are connected to universal power and love, and yet are also separate from society and others or their influence, you are able to function well within it.

Remember a time when you were present: perhaps when you were fully engaged in a riveting conversation with someone who was also present; making love with your beloved partner for the first time or after being apart for so long; connected with nature; anything that made you go, 'Ahh'.

I remember once my cat brought me a mouse. It was alive and unharmed, so I picked it up and went outside. I sat in the full moonlight on the grass and laid out my hand to let it go. I felt so much love and appreciation that it was still alive.

Instead of rushing off, it sat on my hand, unfurled itself and looked right at me. I gasped in delight.

He walked up my arm and sat on my shoulder, my head was turned so I could look him in the eyes. Those beautiful big black eyes twinkling, my heart filled with the wonder of nature and love for this being and gratitude for this sacred moment; this true connection.

He saw me and I saw him.

Then he started washing, like a cat does, behind his huge round ears, oh, so cute, I'm sure he did it just to make me mush even more. I talked to him, he continued, no fear in him as there was only awe in me.

At some point, he walked calmly down my arm and turned around to look at me, then slowly walked off. After a few metres, he stopped, turned around and got on his two feet holding his paws up, staring at me, and then he scurried off.

I sat there, stunned, yet fully present. I experienced true love and presence in that short while, and I felt so alive, so vibrant, so at peace. It had a huge impact, so much so, that 20 years later, I still recall it and am beaming as I write this.

For you, such a moment could have been: when you witnessed your child being born; when you first got that pet you so wanted and now he or she is in your arms, in your heart; when you hit that perfect ball and won the game; when you focused during your black belt in a martial arts grading and was just in that kata or set of moves; when that boy or girl finally asked you out; your first kiss; being mesmerised watching a butterfly or a ladybird; anything.

For whatever reason, at that moment you were fully present.

I have had so many present moments that now I attract more of them because I expect and want to. The more you connect and are present, the more powerful it becomes.

Start by being present with yourself. Look deeply in the mirror and talk honestly to yourself. Connect to your body and listen.

Do a daily morning meditation and a presence-ritual.

See the meditation section for extra help.

Touching your body often and sending extra love to it also increases presence.

Then practice presence with others. Just be really attentive, listen more, talk less, look them in the eye, smile and generate self-love and presence so it influences your encounter. Self-love is not sexual, it is pure and limitless.

**Presence is a gift to yourself and to others.**

It is the most precious gift you can offer and is free, limitless, and one size fits all.

**Example:** I visited someone in the hospital and there was an elderly lady, 93 in the corner bed, alone, looking sad. I smiled and ensured I was calm within and went over to her and increased my smile, ensuring love was beaming from it and my eyes.

I gently sat next to her. She smiled back. I nodded and introduced myself and asked for her name. 'Hello Bethany, it is awesome to meet you, thank you for letting me sit next to you'. And then she had tears in her eyes, and I took her hand and just held it, that's it, nothing sexual, no ulterior motive, just connection.

She wasn't able to talk much as she was so frail, then the nurse came to plug her into oxygen and I moved away so she could get access, but afterwards, Bethany reached out for my hand, so I held it again and smiled, and after a while, when I thought she was calmer, I beamed and put her hand on her own lap and nodded again.

'It's been a pleasure meeting you Bethany, if you need anything I will be over there with my Mum.' Then I left, gently, being mindful that when in deep conversation, auras meet and brisk movement can be jolting to both parties, especially if the person is frail or poorly.

That's it, nothing major, but I was present, and that means more aware of your environment and any suffering that you may be able to help alleviate.

At times when I was down, a stranger smiled or made conversation with me from a fully present state, and that lifted my spirits.

Never underestimate the power of a smile, a nod, or just acknowledgement.

\* \* \*

## Reconnect Fully With Your Senses

We are such sensual beings.

I don't mean sensual as in sexy, sexual, or attractive.

## What sensual *actually* means is able to use your senses.

When you are aware of all of your senses at once, this creates a sort of ecstasy, a full-body connection and presence.

We have lots of senses (physical and **energetic**/metaphysical), the most common ones are:

*Sight*, eyes, vision, visualisation, third-eye, day-dreaming, **clairvoyance**

*Sound*, ears, hearing, self-talk, thoughts, **clairaudience**

*Touch*, feeling, hands/body/skin, **clairsentience and clairtangency**

*Smell*, fragrances, nose, **clairolfactory/clairsalience/clairscentency**

*Taste*, tongue, food, drink, **clairgustance**

*Intuition*, inner-sense, gut feeling, **6th Sense**

*Knowing*, existence, presence, **claircognizance**

*Emotional,* able to use our feelings/emotions adequately, **clairempathy**

We have senses on the *physical* and **metaphysical** levels, we are fully sensory beings: we are sense-able and sensitive.

You can see with your physical eyes, and you can visualise with your third-eye or see other frequencies with your clairvoyance.

You can hear with your ears, or with your clairaudience, so you can hear with your inner ears, mediumship, hearing your own inner voice, your inner self-talk, your thoughts or voices that are not from the physical realm.

You can touch, feel or sense with your body, skin or hands and you can also feel or sense from your intuition, your gut. You are able to touch or sense other dimensions, trance-mediumship, shamanism, and you can feel other people's emotions or pain either alive or passed.

Clairtangency is slightly different this is when you can read energy or get messages about someone either dead or alive just by touching something associated with them, or them. This is also known as psychometry.

You can smell with your actual nose and with your clairsalience, also known as clairscentency, but I like my own term which is clairolfactory, so you can smell what isn't there but triggered by a memory, by people or other beings resonating at a different frequency.

You can taste with your tongue, but also with your clairgustance, so you can taste what you are not physically eating, sometimes when channelling people who have past they can come through with a strong taste of their favourite food or drink.

You can sense with your gut or get a sense that something isn't right, or which path to follow and this is a mix of the clairs, so let's call it your 6th sense.

You can learn knowledge and you can use your claircognizance which is when you instinctively know something, you don't need proof or faith, you somehow know

You can feel your emotions and able to use them and when you can sense someone else's emotions or feelings whether dead or alive, this is called clairempathic or being an empath. It is similar to clairsentience only perhaps not as strong.

We are physical and metaphysical sensual beings, capable of so much more than what we generally experience currently.

We are all aware of our physical senses and we can all train our metaphysical senses, our Clair-senses. When we read other people who are alive I call this *psychic* and when we read other beings from different dimensions or people who have passed I call this *spiritual or angelic* and when we read nature beings I call this *etheric or working with the Divas.*

We use our meta-senses to communicate with worlds outside of the physical level.

Some people are more adept to certain senses, and others work on using all of them.

Just by reading this, whether you agree or not, whatever emotions it emoted, bringing this to your consciousness has helped awaken all of your senses at all levels.

If you choose to, now you can cultivate this. Your body is capable of so much more. Self-love, self-understanding, and treating yourself right is a journey that will lead you where you want to go.

And the more present you are, the more you will be able to communicate with your body, and hence your bladder.

Presence plays a huge part in bladder health.

To end this chapter with a bit of relevant humour, I read a Christmas card with a picture of *Darth Vader* from *Star Wars* that said:

*I know what you got for Christmas... Because I felt your presents.*

**Let your presence be felt too: it is a gift.**

## Chapter 7 Keynotes

- Our body talks and we need to actively listen to it.

- Practising mirror work helps to better the connection to self.

- We have different senses. Sensual means being able to use them consciously. We have physical and metaphysical senses.

- Being sensual often helps build presence.

- Don't be a swan; allow victimised secrets out of your system.

- Be present more because it is a gift.

- Higher frequencies help lift up the lower ones. Practice presence often.

- We can connect deeper now with our bladder, and all our body.

## Action! Interactive bit, it's your turn:

1. Do the meditations related to this chapter. Get to know your senses.

2. Write in your journal any moments that you remember in your life when you were fully present and how that felt.

3. Write in your own words why these are important: self-love, presence, being authentic and earnest, forgiveness.

4. What is your favourite, or go-to sense? Why?

5. Write down the mirror work phrases that you are going to use and keep a journal about your mirror work journey.

6. What signals have you set up with your bladder?

So, now that we have discovered our full senses and practised the true meaning of sensuality, we go on to a more practical issue of discussing products.

Oh yeah, get your comfy shoes on, we are going exploring.

# CHAPTER 8

# Products

As already mentioned, all the products you use are important. I realise that I repeat myself in this book, it is on purpose to help the information sink in.

Some studies say you need to read or hear the same thing three times to register it, I'm not sure how true that it, but still, repetition is helpful.

We use a lot of products in our daily life, and making some changes may be challenging, so do it at your own pace.

It's simply swapping a brand to a healthier one. It takes effort when you are searching for which brand to buy but after that, it's just shopping.

You buy toothpaste already right? So, it's no big deal to buy a different brand, or make your own, either is fine.

What we put on our skin, breathe into our lungs, or consume, end up in our blood and eventually in our bladder.

**Check out my YouTube channel for free videos of how to make your own stuff and the Products & Services Reference.**

**Note:** beware of clever marketing. Don't be fooled by product labels saying words like 'natural'. Many natural things are toxic to humans.

Arsenic and petrol are natural, but do you want to eat them or smear them on your skin?

So, dig deeper than what they want you to see.

Scrutinise the ingredients and use Google to look up what they are.

If something says *organic* in big writing on the front label, it may not mean what you think. Check the small print on the back, it may be just one ingredient that is organic.

During my training on aloe vera, I came across a common brand that was most deceiving. On the front label in big letters, it said made with *99% organic aloe vera*. In tiny writing on the back label, it said *made with 1% aloe vera of which 99% is certified organic.*

That is *very* different from leading a consumer to believe the whole product is 99% organic and made with aloe vera. The finished product was 99% chemical-laden with 1% natural organic product. The only reason they put it in there was to obey the organic advertising laws, to be able to use the word *organic* to entice customers, just short of false advertising, in my opinion.

The laws for being able to state a product is organic, differs in each country and changes from time to time. In this case, as the product contained some organic aloe, they could advertise it, but still had to disclose what and the percentage of organic material, but that could be in tiny writing anywhere on the bottle.

Marketing and advertising brainwashing techniques is a whole other book, but I did think it deserved at least a mention in this section.

So we have dealt with nutrition and clothing, so now for the breath. Remember what we breathe also affects our health.

**Fresh Air**

Go outside if possible, every morning and take at least 5 deep breaths, being present. Breathe in as much as you can, hold it for a while, and breathe out slowly.

We breathe in oxygen and we breathe out carbon; in with the good and out with bad.

One way to ensure correct deep breathing is to put one hand on your heart and one on your lower belly. When breathing in, your lower hand should move out. It should move in when breathing out. Your top hand should not move. You want to breathe deeply into the lower depths of your lungs, they are huge, so pull air down into the tummy and diaphragm.

Breathe in nature when possible, this adds to the quality and true connection. By the sea, in a forest, in a field, on a glacier, wherever.

Wherever you are, fill up with oxygen deeply so it can reach your cells. The more you breathe with awareness, the more presence you create.

Be mindful of the air quality and take precautions when you can: when filling up with petrol, use the free gloves provided at the pump, a scarf around your face, reducing the fumes you are breathing in; sitting in air conditioning or a plane where the air is polluted with other people's germs, wear a scarf around your nose for some of the time and as soon as you are out, take deep breaths and then exhale all the air, this is to expel any toxins or germs that we recently inhaled. Push them out of your lungs, then deep breaths in again.

Drink plenty of water to help flush out germs from your system; avoid being too close to people who are spluttering and sneezing; if in your car and in traffic or near roadworks, put the button on so that only air in the car circulates, not pulling in air from outside; avoid harsh nasal sprays, use home-made ones with water with salt or buy ready-made saline water; keep your airways clear and clean, but not laden with chemicals or irritants; hold your breath passing perfume counters; or if still using aerosol deodorants, although by the end of this chapter, I hope you won't be any more.

Proper breathing is important for bladder health.

* * *

So, we have already discussed what we put in our mouth in previous chapters; food, drink, nail-biting and other body parts.

Now, let's talk about what we put on our skin or what we touch, and let's make it clear again that *anything* touching your skin will impact your health.

Over time we build up a tolerance to these toxins, but that's not a good thing; it means our bodies have got used to a bad situation.

## Products to look out for:

### Laundry

Washing powders or liquids. Most commercial products will have harsh chemicals and fake fragrances.

For the last 12 years, I use an aloe vera multi-purpose cleanser.

Recently, I also make my own using soap nuts. I place 8 soap nuts in a small cotton bag (it comes free with the 1kg bag of soap nuts) and put that directly in the washing machine with the laundry. I use the same little bag of nuts several times.

Soap nuts are natural hard fruits from a tree containing natural saponin, which is a safe cleanser.

For fabric conditioner, I use white vinegar with a few drops of organic lavender oil.

Boom: awesome result and is skin, human and pet-friendly.

### Clothing materials

What clothing is made with is important as this touches your skin for a prolonged time. Most commercial clothing will have nasties in it such as polyester, cheap chemical-laden cotton and toxic dyes.

When possible, buy clothing made from organic natural materials, such as organic cotton, organic hemp, organic linen, organic bamboo, or organic wool.

Now, for the clothing themselves. The most important clothing affecting your bladder health is your knickers, as they touch your precious holes.

My advice is to not wear any. Go 'commando' when you can, and sleep naked.

Your lady-bits need relief from clothing. If you do wear knickers, then treat yourself to some organic cotton ones with a generous gusset.

Never wear strings, thongs or pretty little lacy things, as they gather sweat, candida, germs, pee, poo, and smear up your holes.

Thongs are cystitis waiting to happen, not to mention a cheese-slicer for your butt-crack. Irritation all around, they are a definite no-no.

Organic underwear is not easy to find, so just ensure at least the gusset is pure cotton or bamboo.

Bed Sheets are important as your skin touches those for hours too. Opt for organic cotton or organic bamboo, and clean them often with approved washing products.

## In the bathroom

Scrutinise your body wash, soap, bubble bath, shampoo, conditioner, toothpaste, mouthwash, teeth whitening, floss, moisturisers, body cream, hair mousse, hairsprays, hair dyes, deodorant, hand and foot creams, face creams, toners, make-up, make-up remover, perfumes, body sprays, and aftershave. They all count.

Read labels, read up on company ethics, where they source their raw materials, and if they condone animal testing.

Most commercial products will have nasties including plastics, chemicals, dyes, heavy metals, scents, toxins; things that have no business touching your skin.

The rule is if you wouldn't eat it or put in your mouth, then you should not put it on your skin either.

That may be difficult to do all the time in this toxic society, but do what you can, I call it applying damage limitation.

I avoid fem-washes and douches as they are good marketing ploys but do not help and could make things worse, that is my experience with trying several of these.

The only soap to use near your bits would be one you've tried, tested, and trust and follow with a good rinsing.

## Make-Up

I have mentioned before the potential nasties in make-up so be mindful of where you get yours from, research, read ingredients, and ask the company if need be.

I was horrified in what goes into commercial and even expensive cosmetics, so I stopped wearing make-up until I found a natural one made from primarily aloe vera and went on extensive training with them.

I now also use another brand for makeup. Metaphysics helped me find them. On my way to a self-development convention, I informed the universe that I needed a new makeup range to use and share in my book. There was a stall for natural make-up. I spoke to the CEO and tried the products over the weekend and purchased a bag full. I love them. So now I'm working on getting a discount for my readers whilst I continue using them to ensure they are good enough. Once I do, I'll share it on social media.

Look for the most natural make-up available. Don't be fooled if you pay more for cosmetics, the type you get in salons, 'the posh brands', they have just as many nasties in them if not more; you pay for the name. Beware of marketing.

In my training, I came across an article explaining that surgeons removed lumps of plastic from ladies' under eyes before doing liftings, because they had used eye-creams, even really expensive brands for years, thinking they were doing themselves a good service. The polymers (plastic) in the cream eventually clumped together under the skin and formed plastic balls. So, if you use eye cream, beware to use a natural one, as much as possible.

Remember your skin quality depends mainly on your nutrition and hydration, so get that right and your skin will be healthy and glow without any external products.

Beauty comes from within.

## Animal Cruelty in Any Products

I did warn you this book would get deep and approach taboo subjects. I like to keep my promises.

Any product we put on our skin or pay money for will influence our energetic health. If an animal has suffered to make your product – tested on, abused, beaten, killed, crushed up as an ingredient, turned into a fur coat – then those low frequencies will be in the product, and then into you.

No more ignorance, no more funding abuse of any kind. Vote with your money and value your health above all else. We change the world one person at a time. Refuse to buy these products, and soon these industries will have to stop using and testing on animals, and stop slave labour and unethical behaviour to make a quick buck.

They are interested in profit and selling their product, and that is fine, that is what all companies need, but there are ethical ways to do that and with fewer pollutants that harm us, the animals, the plants, food sources, air quality, and the planet.

Support companies that do that already, even if it means paying more.

Please consider being this person, and take back your power from the big industries, governments, and marketing campaigns.

Please be that person who stands up for animals and the planet and for yourself.

I do sometimes make my own toothpaste with organic coconut oil, bicarbonate of soda and organic essential oil of peppermint and tea tree.

Be aware most kinds of toothpaste have fluoride. This is not good for our teeth like most in the dental industry say. I know hundreds of people that use fluoride-free toothpaste, myself included for the last 12 years, and have awesome teeth.

So, please avoid fluoride, sugars, sweeteners, and alcohol in your toothpaste.

I now also use organic coconut oil as a body and face moisturiser and hair mask.

Sometimes, but rarely as it is a palaver, I make my own shampoo and body wash using the soap nuts. Boil them for 30 mins, let cool, whizz up the water in a blender, it makes a sumptuous silky foam and use right away.

I sometimes also use this liquid to do the washing up with and then re-use the cooked nuts for my laundry.

A great homemade shampoo is bicarbonate of soda powder massaged on wet hair, then rinse.

Then pour on neat organic apple cider vinegar, leave for a few minutes then rinse, it is an awesome de-tangler and conditioner.

## Hair Dyes

It took me a long time to find a hair dye that was natural and that I was happy with. So beware, commercial hair dyes are toxic and what goes on

your scalp ends up in your body I have a link to them in the Products &
Services Reference.

I know we want to look our best, so I'm not saying to never dye your
hair, I'm saying be mindful and look into better choices. The best natural
hair dye that I have found that works really well and is good for you and
healthy, is a good quality henna brand.

So, safe dye is the way forward, especially if you are someone who colours
their hair regularly, I know some who go to the hairdressers every 6 weeks
for a trim and colour, imagine the levels of toxins your liver and whole
body needs to clear to have coloured hair, there are good alternatives out
there.

**Nail Varnish/Polish**

OK, there aren't any, that I have found, that are non-toxic. So be aware
that yes, what goes on your nails will end up in your body, and if you are
someone that bites your nails, minute particles of it will also get in your
mouth and down your throat, along with any nasties living under your
nails or around your fingers.

I love long coloured nails and I do sometimes let them grow and have
them manicured with a bright polish and that is OK, because it is my
choice, and I ensure my hygiene is top-notch by using a natural nail
brush and my aloe vera soap.

And I give my nails a break from varnish for most of the year.

Formaldehyde is used in nail varnish/polish. Formaldehyde is a
carcinogen.

**Period Products**

I haven't used tampons since one gave me cystitis and since my research informed me that some tampons have harsh chemicals inside them and that some women can get life-threatening reactions to them.

That's too high a price to pay for period-mopping.

Tampons also irritate the vagina, are messy to deal with, and not too easy or comfortable to use. I also found that pulling it out irritated my skin, and if one precious hole is inflamed, it may impact the others. There are alternatives.

If you choose to continue using tampons, ensure you change them very regularly and that you have clean hands when you do. Pull the string down or away as you pee to avoid getting that wet, and when you poo, pull the string away so it doesn't get smeared when you wipe your butt, as that string touches your urethra once it's all nestled in your knickers, especially tight knickers or thongs.

The best thing to do is to change your tampon each time you wee or poo.

I don't like most sanitary towels, as they have an irritating material and can be filled with chemicals or plastics. I have used organic cotton pads.

Another good tool to use is a 'Moon-Cup' which is a small rubber cup that you insert into the vagina and the blood collects in there, you pull it out, empty, rinse, and put it back in. It is very economical in the long run and more hygienic than tampons, but it can be quite a palaver whilst getting used to it. I used one for years.

If you use sanitary towels or incontinence pads, change them regularly and don't sit in damp material rubbing for too long on your urethra.

There are also special menstruation or incontinence knickers instead of tampons, towels or moon-cups, but I never tried these and I'm not sure about them as it involves sitting in it all day, as I'm assuming we don't change the knickers in a day?

If you wish to try them let the tribe know how you get on with them but to be clear, I did not try these and even if I did still have periods, I wouldn't bother as I was OK with the organic pads and moon-cup, but I like to keep on top of what is new. I have put further details in the free gift previously mentioned.

## Catheters

If you need one, ensure great hygiene and ask to have your urine dipped regularly to check for infection and check that your urine colour is clear to yellow.
See the catheter tips from Part One.

## Toilet Roll

White cotton is best. Avoid those feminine wet wipes. If you have forgotten your water bottle and flannel to wash your butt with after a poo, and you are not at home able to wash, then yes, do use a wet-wipe for your butt, but not your vagina or urethra.

## Towels/Flannels

Organic cotton, organic hemp or bamboo is best. At the very least, high-quality cotton. Don't leave them on the heated rack because damp towels tend to go hard or smell funny on those. Let them dry naturally in fresh air by an open window. Change them often and ensure they are washed in natural products.

**Jewellery/watches**

If it's gold, silver, wood or stainless steel, then it's fine.

If it's plastic, rubber, cheap metals, or aluminium, then this could cause irritations, and if pierced into the ears, tummy, nipples or clit, then infections are probable.

**Water**

Golden rule: if it isn't safe to drink, it isn't safe to bathe in.

You may get away with showering in it, providing you don't aim the shower directly up to your precious holes, but since getting really bad cystitis after bathing in dirty water, I now rinse my bits with mineral water if I'm abroad in a country where I don't trust the water.

Even at home, I use a filtering shower head making my water for showering a little less harsh, and I have one that fits around my bath tap for baths, but this won't make the water drinkable or clean enough to bathe in, if it isn't already potable.

**Note:** Jacuzzi and most swimming pools are loaded with high levels of chlorine and other chemicals that irritate your precious holes, but it may be preferable to the myriad of germs. Ensure proper hygiene before and after using these.

This environment is irritating to your precious holes and can be a cystitis trigger.

Avoid sex in the pool, Jacuzzi, the sea, or bath or shower. Yes, it may seem romantic but opening up precious holes whilst submerged means anything in that water will travel up your vagina (into the womb) your anus (into the colon) and of course your precious urethra (into the bladder).

## Shoes

Yes, they do play a small part, but not so much as we usually wear socks, again organic cotton or bamboo socks would be ideal.

It is OK to wear shoes for bladder health, but I'm being thorough and over-delivering on my promise to share as much information as possible within a bladder book.

So, make sure you are comfortable in your shoes, not too tight, fully supported and cushioned, avoid high heels as this affects your posture and your balance and so potentially may affect your bladder health, not to mention your back and chances of falling over.

If you have correct footwear or are barefooted, you can stand and breathe better and so your bladder is well oxygenated and supported in the correct position, it is not hunched over, trying to hold itself up or pushing too hard on the vaginal walls.

## Perfumes, Aftershave

I haven't found any that do not contain alcohol or nasties, so use whatever you want, but spray less and spray it on your clothing, not on your skin and avoid breathing in whilst you spray. Be aware as you become less toxified you may be more sensitive and less tolerant of other people's perfumes or sprays.

## Deodorants and Antiperspirants

Avoid aerosols. Avoid aluminium salts. Most will have those highly toxic chemicals that are linked to breast cancer amongst other nasties. Antiperspirants block your pores and this means not only are you adding directly near your lymph nodes (armpits) toxins and cancer-causing chemicals, but you are also closing off the pores so that your body cannot sweat them or other toxins out.

Oh, no, not on my watch: it's time to stop using commercial deodorants and especially antiperspirants.

I use an aloe vera stick and it works brilliantly, and it's safe.

You can use rock salt or other natural ones, but I found they did not work so well.

Whichever one you decide to use, make sure it does not contain aluminium as that is crucial. Beyond that, it is also best to avoid polymers (plastics), alcohol, sugar, but the main thing is no aluminium. I can't stress that enough.

## Household

What do you clean your house with, floors, surfaces, mantelpiece, furniture, sink, washing-up? All of these will affect your health. You touch it, sit on it, and breathe it in, and so do your children and pets.

Once you get more present and connected with your body, it will tell you it doesn't like things that before you were unaware of. Your senses will heighten, and you will become less tolerant of pollutants, and that is a good thing.

There are many safe natural products available now, I have tried many and some work better than others, and some are more expensive.

For all house-cleaning, I use an aloe vera multi-purpose cleanser or make my own.

You decide what works best for you.

**Example:** If I wash up at my mum's using a standard washing up liquid, my throat clams up, my nostrils itch, I get a slight headache, and feel a bit sick. That is normal because the chemicals and artificial scents in these products are irritants to the skin and pollutants to our airways.

Aloe vera or soap-nuts are versatile and can wash anything and are safe for pets too. The advantage is that fleas and mosquitos do not like aloe vera, so it is a natural antimicrobial anti-insect too, great to wash your pet or pet bedding. I have used this to clean my sofa and carpets too.

Experiment, play and investigate for yourself.

I also sometimes make my own cleaning products for the house using bicarbonate of soda, white vinegar and lemon.

See my YouTube channel for free info on how I use the products or make my own.

Use neat bicarbonate as laundry powder, mix it with water for cleaning surfaces or pans, add lemon or vinegar to make it fizz, and degrease.

So to recap, there are many brands that are more natural or organic and less toxic to use on our body, clothes, and house, and there are lots of ways of making your own products too.

You do not need to rely on standard commercial products anymore that are damaging to your health, especially as you come into contact with them or in the air on a daily basis, so this adds to the continuous compound impact.

Be mindful of all the products you choose to use.

**Tattoos**

Oh my, yes I'm over-delivering, but hey, with good information: more is more.

I love tattoos, but be mindful of the ink, it is a foreign substance forced into your skin and may be toxic. Take your time choosing the tattoo artist, their level of hygiene, and look into what ink they use, some are safer than others.

And take care to treat yourself well to ensure quick hygienic healing.

**Top tip:** I used a high-quality aloe vera gel drink, aloe vera and propolis cream, and this is my successful tattoo story: I drank lots of aloe vera the day before and on the day itself. I brought in a bottle of it with a straw (as I was lying down) and I sipped the whole thing (1 litre) by the time we were done. I was in the chair for 8 hours, so there was no need to gulp it fast. Once home, I used aloe vera soap and pat dry with a clean organic cotton towel and then lathered on the aloe vera gel and then at night I used the aloe & propolis cream.

Two days later I went back for the tattoo artist to check the development and he was shocked, stating I had over 1 week worth of improvement in less than two days, and what was my secret.

It does make a difference using great products when your body really needs it and having a tattoo, especially large ones, is traumatic for your whole system.

And remember, a tattoo is for life. Metaphysically, what is on your skin and exposed to the world is also in your aura and forms part of your frequency.

So make sure it is a tattoo that you love and brings you joy, not sadness because that will forever contribute to your energy frequency. I don't regret any of mine, they all mean something magical to me, and I smile when I see them.

### Cookware and Food Containers

What touches your food touches you. So be mindful of food wrapped in plastic or in tins, cans are usually aluminium, which is toxic for human well-being.

Of course, sometimes even wild or organic food comes wrapped, but many companies now are more environmentally friendly and choose bamboo, cardboard or paper with a renewable tree scheme for food preparation and delivery.

You can control how you store your own food. Avoid cling-film or tin foil.

I use glass containers to store my food. I eat from glass, crockery or bamboo, not plastic or tin.

How you cook your food is important. I avoid copper, aluminium, tin, all non-stick, Teflon, silicon or plastics.

Unless you want highly toxic, dead, nuclear non-food, then never use a microwave.

I repeat, do not use microwaves. What you gain in convenience, you lose in health.

I cook in stainless steel, glass or cast-iron pans.

My utensils are stainless steel or bamboo.

\* \* \*

Part of my work is to do health talks and in the past, I used to present some products. I heard the excuse so many times, 'I can't afford good products', and some even said that before knowing the prices!

We are programmed to think poor, to have a lack-belief, but in reality, think of it like this:

I asked those who said they can't afford better products what they did spend money on, what they could afford beyond the basics, what I class as a luxury.

For example: did they have coffee most days from a coffee shop? Most said yes, and it cost about £3, sometimes they have a muffin with it and it then costs about £7, so an average £4.50 on coffee shops per day.

Did they park in town daily and pay instead of parking further away for free, or walk, take the bus, or cycle? Most did park, yes, another £2 to £25 depending on the length of stay.

Do they eat lunch out most days or buy it and eat at their desk instead of making their own from home? Some said yes, costing about £10 for lunch.

Do they go to the pub, how much do they spend there every weekend, or daily?

Do they smoke, how much is their tobacco habit costing them per week?

Do they play the lottery, if so how many tickets?

Do they buy the expensive drinks, popcorn, sweets, or ice cream at the cinema?

Do they brush their teeth, use shampoo, etc..? Yes, and the money they spent on them depended on the brand.

You get the idea.

Add up all the 'luxury' stuff they are willing to pay for, and then realise that they are spending money without thinking, and could easily make savings.

If they brought coffee from home in stainless-steel flask it would save approx. £4 per day. Making their own lunch by bringing in leftovers, or their own food they have prepared would save between £5 and £10 per day.

Parking further away, using public transport, or walking when possible saves heaps of money. And if we deduct what they already pay for their products or clothing anyway from what a good, organic brand costs, they only need to cover the *difference* to treat themselves well.

The point is that most people can afford organic and planet-friendly food, products and clothing, but they choose not to and hide behind not affording it.

Maybe some truly can't afford the difference as their lifestyle stands, but if prepared to make small daily changes, they might. It just depends on where you value your money. It could be some really can't afford it, and that's OK, they can still just employ damage limitations where possible.

I don't spend much money at coffee shops. I don't always park in central town where parking fees are ludicrous anyway. I don't pay the cinema food prices. I don't drink much alcohol and not in pubs. I choose not to smoke. I don't play the lottery. Those choices save me lots of money so I can spend more on what I value.

I value good-energy people and animal-friendly products, clothing, and food, when available.

I'm not saying you have to, I'm explaining that being truthful, and not making excuses, is the A-Team way.

Remember that authenticity is important for bladder health, self-love and self-valuing. Are you and your body not worth the best fuel and products?

Before stating that you can't afford organic, or better brands, ask yourself if that is *strictly* true.

What do you spend money on that is not health-promoting or that you could cut back on but don't?

Where could you make changes so that you could afford to treat yourself better?

I use an aloe and propolis tooth gel retailing at approximately £6 a tube. The cheapest toothpaste is about £2 and the average is about £3. I make that choice because I can't honestly say that I can't afford an extra couple of pounds to treat my body and the planet right. I'm not lining pockets of abusers with my choice.

I'm not eating fluoride that is chronically intoxicating my system twice a day.

**So there you are. I have shared what I use for my products, a mix of:**

- Bicarbonate of Soda

- White vinegar

- Organic Apple Cider Vinegar

- Organic Wax-Free Lemons

- Organic coconut oil

- Organic Essential Oils

- Soap Nuts

- Henna

- High-Quality Aloe Vera

To conclude this section, homemade products is the A-Game as you can source raw materials that are organic, cruelty-free with happy vibes, and make up the products to use yourself.

Second is best is to buy products that are the healthiest for your skin and a brand with high ethics and completely animal and human-friendly.

## Chapter 8 Keynotes

- What we put on our skin affects our well-being.

- Avoid harsh chemicals in products. Some of the worst are aluminium, fluoride, aspartame, lead, mercury, plastics.

- Ensure a product is truly animal-friendly. The energetic frequencies of products affect our well-being too.

- Make your own products using soap-nuts, bicarbonate of soda, vinegar, and organic coconut oil.

- Find a brand that you love and trust.

- Details of the products, cookware and clothing I use can be found in the Products & Services Reference, the link to which is part of your free gifts at the front of this book.

## Action! Interactive bit, it's your turn:

1. Put all of your current products, if not already natural, in a box in the garage. You can return to them after your adventure if you still want them.

2. Find a brand that works for you, it doesn't have to be totally organic or natural but do ensure it is energetically clean and that they do not contain the worst of the toxins or abused animals.

3. Now use that brand, or make your own during the 8 weeks of cleanout. It is time to clean up your skin, body, and environment by using safer products for everything.

4. After using these for a while, get out your old products and use those for one day. Really pay attention to your body's reactions.

What are your senses telling you? Is your nose twitching at the smell? Do you feel a little nauseous? Is your skin recoiling or itchy, sensitive? Does your scalp burn a little? Do your teeth feel tighter or your mouth slightly swollen?

Do your clothes smell fake? What is your intuition saying? Truly notice all the signs. Either put the old products back in the garage for future use or give them away to someone who is not bothered about chemicals or recycle them.

5.  Access the *Products & Services Reference* (drjmeyer.com/free-gifts) for specific details of what I use.

6.  Go to my YouTube channel (youtube.com/channel/UCVHKRGdC7twLEVVIUMhkkxQ) to see how I make my own products.

This concludes our products section.

I hope it has been useful. You can kick off your shoes and chill out now.

When you are ready, I'll meet you in the next chapter, it's all about community.

## CHAPTER 9

# Building Hope & Your True Tribe

Remember that story of 'monkey see, monkey do', that who you spend most of your time with (virtually, in person, or in books) will contribute to your character, choices in life, and your personal frequency and hence what you attract?

It's time to pay attention to who you hang around with. To have good bladder health, hang around with healthy people who practice the protocols in this book, who, like you, are putting their health and well-being as a priority in life.

Hang around with people hungry for self-development and finding ways to increase their life quality and quantity.

Those who light you up, not bring you down.

Those who encourage you, not jealous of your accomplishments.

Those who celebrate with you, not talk behind your back or ignore you.

Those who practice self-love and presence or at least, are on that journey.

You get the idea.

Be mindful of social decluttering; make room in your life for your true tribe.

Form the community you want to flourish in.

**Who are you real monkeys?**

There are many ways you can do that. Read books that inspire you, see who else has read them and converse about them, share more ideas. You could even start your own book club in your area.

Go to workshops and classes that inspire you. Attending self-development retreats or classes and events that interest you, gives you the opportunity to meet people you have common interests with.

Go to conventions that appeal to you and talk to people, swap details, and stay in touch. I love going to writers' festivals or metaphysical conferences for that reason.

It also keeps me on my toes and helps my continuous research of what's new in fields that I'm interested in and want to write about.

What can you do to increase your true tribe?

**To see the importance of building a happy network and true tribes, see my '*Acknowledgments*' page at the end of this book.**

If you haven't yet done so then join 'The Happy Bladder Tribe', the Facebook group. In this group you can breathe, it is a safe space with no judgement.

The more you teach and share, the more it helps you, so this community is about you.

Please come in and tell your story, ask for help, offer help, the more you get involved in it, the more you will get out of it.

It is also useful as reminders of what the book is about. Someone may share about a protocol success story, reminding you that you haven't adopted that protocol yet.

It will be like mini-repetitions of useful information.

Stand up for yourself and don't let any cystitis taboos or embarrassment stop you from speaking out or doing what it takes to avoid it.

Another potential way to increase your tribe is to join a network marketing company whose products and ethics you love. When I did, I had access to some like-minded people and fun training. I had the opportunity to go for incentives that resulted in me going abroad & the UK for rallies. Just to be clear, the incentives are earned, and being a distributor is not a paid job, it is a business that you need to work hard at.

## Further Hope

There is further help coming aside from this book and the tribe as in 2020 I will be focusing on the *Piss to Bliss Movement*.

I will be creating the following:

- In-depth, hand-holding online course on bladder health

- shorter Facebook challenges on the matter

- publishing *Piss to Bliss Companion* to really help you whilst reading this book again, each time you go on this journey you will find another piece of gold.

- publishing a version & companion for girls or peeps who do not want any swearing or who are no longer sexually active, *called Yip-Pee & Yip-Pee Pal*

- doing public talks, especially in the USA and the UK, about bladder health.

- There is also talk (in my head) of a retreat where a few of us get pampered for a week in a rural French house really digging deep on transforming our bladder health at all levels.

So you are not alone.

We've got this.

If you wish to be kept informed of future events or books then look out for announcements in the Facebook Tribe and also subscribe to our newsletter.

You can do that by entering your email on our website www.drjmeyer.com

## Chapter 9 Keynotes

- 'Monkey see monkey do', who you spend your time with will influence you.

- There is hope for living cystitis-free.

## Action! Interactive bit, it's your turn:

1. Join our community Facebook group and introduce yourself.

2. Write in your journal anything or anyone that you feel is no longer good for your health or to hang around with. What glimmers of hope do you have now?

3. Write in your journal fun ways you are going to increase your positive community.
   What does your true tribe look like?

So, now that we have enhanced hope that help and support are there, we flow blissfully to the next chapter, entering the magical realm of meditation.

# CHAPTER 10

# Meditations

I created my own meditations to help you with your bladder health quest.

Feel free to use any meditation that you love or are attracted to; there are plenty to download from the internet or to buy on CD.

I have designed these specifically for this book, so do give them a try, even if you feel silly at first.

Come on in, metaphysics is a world of fun and magic.

To really enjoy these meditations, read them through first, then record yourself slowly reading them out loud, and then listen to your own voice guiding you.

If you have earphones and store the file on your mobile phone, you can meditate with them anytime, anyplace but not whilst driving or walking around.

The meditation will work just as well without the voice recording, read it through once, and then again to remember the steps, then close your eyes and do it.

**Note**: do not read or listen to the meditations whilst driving, walking, cycling, operating machinery, or handling sharp objects. For meditations to be truly powerful, it's best to dedicate quality time to them and be present.

1. Meditation to meet your bladder and make that deep connection.

2. Meditation creating communication with your bladder to set up a signal system.

3. Meditation as a daily morning ritual tuning into the right frequency for the day.

4. Meditation as an emergency SOS rescue mission for when you have cystitis: the reset button.

5. Meditation specifically for bladder-cancer sufferers.

**Note:** If you are not able to stand or lie down for any reason, all meditations can be adapted to however you can be comfortable. If you are not able to move your arms or legs, close your eyes and visualise yourself standing in the sunshine or starlight.

So if I say something that you are not physically able to do, please adapt the instruction so that you can follow.

Please, don't worry, positions are just suggestions, pick one that suits you.

The same goes with protocols, if physically you are unable to do some, adapt where possible, there is always a way.

In my meditations, I sometimes use nouns instead of adjectives or verbs. What I mean by that is, for example, I say 'I am presence' instead of 'I am present'. 'I am love' instead of 'I am loved' and 'I am powerful, or I am power', instead of 'I have power'. This is on purpose. I find that it gives the sentence more power.

What I call 'powerful phrases' are also known as positive affirmations or mantras. Our subconscious plays a huge role in manifesting, and the stronger our affirmations the more powerful they are. If we say 'I am loved', there is an underlying voice that says, therefore, I can also *not* be loved.

If we say 'I have power, I have money', it also denotes we may lose it. Therefore if we *are* the thing, it becomes part of our identity and not a possession or temporary thing. We can't lose who we are unless we decide to change. Therefore *I am love* is a stronger frequency than *I am loved*.

\* \* \*

## Meditation 1: Meet your Bladder

Stand straight with good posture and take three deep breaths in and slowly out.

Imagine your feet growing roots, connecting deeply in the ground, reaching the centre of the Earth. Feel that nurturing pulse and see her energy coming up the roots into your feet, up your spine, arms, and head, then cascading out from your crown and falling back through your aura into the ground and back up your feet again.

Put your hands up to the sky, stretch and smile. Imagine your hands cupping the centre of the sun and feel that regenerative solar power pulsing down your hands, arms, head, and down your body, out of your feet, and back up through your aura returning to the sun and back down to you.

Enjoy being totally earth and solar-powered.

You are feeling truly connected and safe.

Breathe in to the count of 6, hold it for 5, and release it slowly for a count of 7.

Bring down your hands and place your palms on your lower belly over your bladder.

If you haven't done so yet, please close your eyes, and release your neck so you can rest your chin down if you wish. Ensure your head is comfortable and your spine is stretched, your chakras are neatly stacked on top of each other and your meridians are relaxed, as good posture will help energise you and ensure that your bladder is in the right position.

Really feel your full presence in your body, no matter what condition your body is in, or what position you are in. Feel the gratitude for your body, what it does for you. Be thankful it is still here for you under whatever circumstance, still willing to be your best friend.

Feel the love of the earth and the sun supporting you.

Feel the energy in your palms warming up, as this wonderful grounded energy is gathering in them and seeping into your skin and through your abdomen. Now start following that flow of energy.

You can pretend you are a tiny person in a blue submarine with large glass windows, flowing in the energy from your hands into the belly.

Keep going until you feel the silky spongy wall and a cave opens up, allowing you into the bladder, a clean and quiet cave.

Look out of your submarine and notice how clear the water is, the visibility is magnificent, and this whole place feels safe, and it is just for you. It is your own private underwater cave.

In this wonderful place, you can breathe easily underwater, so if you choose to, you can leave your submarine, in full scuba gear if you prefer, or naked. If you rather stay in your submarine, you can use that to explore too.

Have a real good gander.

I invite you now to swim or sail right in front of you, until you reach the wall, notice that gorgeous surface, beautiful skin-coloured wall pulsing with vibrancy and healthy vibes. It is joyful and ready to serve.

Swim around the wall, notice it forms a large circle; you are inside a round haven, which is delighted by your visit.

All the walls are clean and vibrate warmly at your presence.

You find a tube, and fresh water is falling through it into the vibrant sea within the cave. And you notice there is another one on the opposite side of the sphere, also splashing. Take a while to enjoy being here and explore these glorious waterfalls.

Now, something amazing happens. So, you get back into your submarine and face downward with the lights shining on this fun event.

Water starts to swirl as a hole unfurls.

The opening gets wider and the water gathers up swirling excitedly, pouring itself down this tube. You are bouncing on the top of the swirl.

As you go down with the water, you notice the cave walls are drying up and start to fold up twisting into a tight ball. As the levels keep going down, the cave disappears.

You now approach the tube opening, and along with the last drops of the water, you enter the tunnel; whoosh, down you go, laughing joyfully, like in a water slide at a theme park. You giggle and enjoy the ride. It is a freeing experience, all the way down, splish, splash and splosh.

You see a light rapidly appear and whoosh, you are now out of the tube and flying in the fresh air, you look back and the beautiful opening just as the tube squeezes shut and disappears.

You gently ride the last wave into your submarine base. You are clean and safe.

You leave your submarine and float back into your body.

Now, reach up to the sky again and connect once more to the sun. Push on your feet to feel the bounce of the earth as you enjoy her energies holding you.

As you take a deep breath, pull your hands down to your heart and breathe out.

You are full of gratitude for what your bladder does for you and thankful that you have this connection.

Take a deep breath and slowly open your eyes.

Smile, you have now made a deep connection with your bladder, ureters and urethra, and all is well. Recognise that your bladder's happiness and ability to serve you properly is all in your hands.

Congratulations, you have met your new best friend.

* * *

## Meditation 2: Setting Up Signals with Your Bladder

This is a team meeting between you (your conscious and subconscious) and your bladder, to set up a signal system so that your bladder can inform you right away if it needs anything.

Ready? Let's dive.

Stand straight with good posture and take three deep breaths in and slowly out.

Imagine your feet growing roots connecting deeply in the ground, reaching the centre of the Earth. Feel that nurturing pulse coming up the roots into your feet, up your spine, arms and head, then cascading out from your crown and falling back through your aura into the ground and back up your feet again.

Put your hands up to the sky, stretch and smile. Imagine your hands cupping the centre of the sun. Feel that powerful solar power pulsing down your hands, arms, head, and down your body, out of your feet and back up through your aura returning to the sun and back down to you.

Enjoy being totally earth and solar-powered.

You are feeling truly connected and safe.

Breathe in to the count of 5, hold it for 5, and release it slowly for 6.

Bring down your hands and place your palms on your lower belly over your bladder area, and breathe normally.

If you haven't done so yet, please close your eyes, and release your neck so you can rest your chin down if you wish. Ensure your head is comfortable but your spine is stretched, your chakras are well stacked and your meridians relaxed.

A good posture will help energy flow and your bladder sit in the right position.

Really feel your full presence in your body. No matter what condition your body is in, what position you are in. Right now, feel the gratitude for your body, what it does for you. Be thankful that it's still here for you under whatever circumstance, willing to be your best friend.

Feel the love of the earth and the sun supporting you.

From this space of peace, truly increase your presence in your body.

Feel the energy in your palms warming up as this wonderful grounded magic is gathering in them and seeping into your skin and your abdomen.

Follow this energy permeating into your bladder.

Notice all your body sensations as you connect to the bladder.

What can you touch, sense or feel, is it warm, tingling, pulsing, a vibrancy?

What can you feel on your body? What does your skin sense, cold, warm, air circulation, clothing resting on it?

Can you feel the security of the ground under your feet?

Take a deep breath, what can you smell? How does that air feel like in your nostrils as it goes deep into your lungs?

Swallow, what can you taste? What does your mouth tell you?

Listen, what sounds can you hear? How near is it? Now zone further out, what noises are far away? What about closer still, what can you hear inside your own body?

Perhaps your pulse, possible shuffling, or your breath, your thoughts?

Just observe, becoming more and more present.

What can you see? Open your eyes, what colours, shapes? Now, close your eyes again, what can you observe with eyes closed? Darkness, light, shapes, sensation of colours, filaments swimming around? Perhaps images of the underwater cave?

What does your intuition tell you? Your inner sense, your 6th sense, your gut?

You are now in this place of acknowledgement, presence, and in tune with your senses. Be here and now. You are fully present and sensual.

Enjoy being with yourself. This is precious quality time between you and your body and the marvels that you are.

Take another deep breath and now put all of your sensual attention into your bladder and settle there for a while.

Let your bladder know you have arrived; you are fully present with all your senses in the centre of your bladder. You are ready to have this important meeting.

Grounded and fully connected, we start the meeting. Trust that the bladder knows what it needs. Trust you are a brilliant team and fully prepared, perhaps with power-point presentations. Your bladder has been waiting for this meeting for a long time.

Now, you have shown up, so be the gift it has been waiting for. All it wants is your understanding and knowledge of what it needs for you to make the best decisions on what to eat, drink, breathe and make lifestyle choices that harmonise with your bladder. Its goal is to keep you healthy and happy, and you have to provide it with what it needs to do that.

This meeting is officially in session.

Notice which of your senses is the strongest right now in your bladder.

Can you really see yourself in your bladder, talking? At this point, you can have a representative of your bladder and yourself show up around the meeting table. They can be any form, colour, anything is fine, and whichever way your bladder wishes to represent itself, let it be. And don't worry if nothing comes, it is still working.

So, what can you see? It could be the bladder itself, a representative, or even the cave we explored in the first meditation.

Look around the chosen meeting room.

What can you observe?

What does your bladder sound like? Ask him to speak to you. It could be a song, a tune, a sound, or a voice, anything is fine, just notice what sounds are present now in the bladder.

What does it feel like? Touch your bladder walls, shake hands or hug the representative.

How does your body react to being in your bladder? What does your inner sense, your intuition and your gut, whilst present within your bladder, tell you?

How does it feel to be intuitively connected to your bladder?

Is there a smell here, what scent does your bladder have right now? It may be something you are not expecting, like roses, chocolate, cut-grass or nothing. Whatever it is, simply observe and be with it, no judgement, don't try and change it. All is fine.

From this present state, sit at the conference table and speak.

'Hello, bladder. I am here. As you know, this meeting is for us to set up a signal system, so that consciously you can talk to me and I can check in with you at any time. Please, let me know when you are starting to be in troubled waters so that I can help you before you get full-blown cystitis.

We also need to set up a proper alarm signal for when it is too late and you are already poorly. What I can do to help you. And to set up a signal just to appease me and tell me that all is well. Whichever signals work for you is perfect, and know we can always change the signals at a later date.'

Smile and wait for an acknowledgement from your bladder.

You will know the signal.

It could be a visual signal. Such as setting up your beach scene; your subconscious as the lifeguard on his white tower looking out to the calm ocean. The ocean is your happy bladder, and there is a flagpole and the flag is currently green, signalling that all is well.

There is an orange flag to signal something is amiss and to pay attention and take precautions.

There is a red flag for when there is a full-on problem and we need to deploy a rescue team and weather the storm.

All flags are on standby for the lifeguard to flag up to your consciousness.

If you prefer hearing the message, then set up a sound alarm system. You can pretend you are in a recording studio or it can be a simple orchestra, or even simpler still, an alarm sound.

Ask your bladder which sound it wants to represent that all is well, it could be a gently little ding. If something is starting to brew, it could be a loud crash, and if something is really bad, it could be a loud bang. Whichever sound is fine, as long as it makes sense to you and it is clearly set up between you and your bladder.

Take a deep breath and spend quality time now with your bladder.

Sit together and work properly to set up your 3 signals in whichever way feels right. Make sure the signal is clear.

And know you can come back to this meeting place anytime you like to change signals or just hang out with your bladder's consciousness.

Once you feel the meeting is over, thank your bladder and all involved.

Show your gratitude for all it has done for you. Acknowledge its wars and any scars from any previous cystitis. From now on, things have changed, you are aware of how to keep the bladder happy and fully functional and you are now on its side.

Forgive yourself for your past actions. Take responsibility for your health. Acknowledge it is not your bladder's fault, because *you* chose the drinks, foods, levels of hygiene, and to hang onto things.

Don't blame yourself either as you were not fully aware of your actions or their consequences.

At this point, if energy needs to be released, then let it out. This is deep emotional cleansing. Cry, sob, and let the stories and secrets out, scream, or imagine the blockages released and going down the drain. Do whatever it takes, command that energy frequency to go, as you no longer need it.

Now, we know what we can do, so we can make the best choices for ourselves every day. Awareness is key and you have it, so use it.

Decide to leave the past behind and start fresh. You have a clean slate. From now on, you and your bladder are best friends and an awesome team.

When you feel the air is clear and all is peaceful and there is nothing but love between you and your bladder, then thank it again.

Now, take a deep breath and make a commitment:

Bladder, I commit to you that every day I will make efforts towards your health.

Bladder, I commit to you that I will listen to your signals and hear you when you are in trouble and help you.

Bladder, I commit to you that from now on, we are on the same team.

Bladder, I commit to loving you and treating you with respect.

When you feel that this meeting is over and all is well, take a deep breath and put your hands up to the sky again and stretch high, reaching into the centre of the sun and now bring your hands back to your heart.

Breathe deeply for the count of 7, hold for a count of 6 and release for 7.

Breathe normally. Slowly open your eyes, and smile.

Congratulations you have just taken a major metaphysical step toward working with your bladder and being present. This is marvellous.

\* \* \*

## Meditation 3: Daily Bliss Connection

This is a quick morning ritual to set yourself up for the day in the highest frequency so you can attract likeness in energy: blissful, hopeful, present and healthy.

If possible, make it a routine to do this outside in the morning, barefoot on the grass. Indoors is fine too, maybe as soon as you get out of bed, but the sooner the better. Make a commitment to yourself to do it every morning and it will soon become a habit, just like brushing your teeth.

You can spend as long or as little as you like in this meditation, adding bits to it from other practices or just as it is; it is all good.

Sometimes, I spend way longer doing this, as I like basking in the glow of gratitude. I will speak out lots of reasons why I'm grateful and thank the universe for my life, in detail.

Sometimes, I want to do more breathing exercises and incorporate some yoga movements. Other times, I just do the minimum, connecting up and get the job done quickly.

Each time may be different and that is OK. Remember the more you meditate and are aware of your body, presence and basic metaphysics, the quicker you will change.

Your frequency will resonate higher and so the world will start to look different. People will start noticing that you are different. You will naturally gravitate towards frequencies (people, situations, books, information, food, hobbies and so forth) that vibrate at a higher frequency and are healthier. This is all part of your journey.

**Here we go, let us begin:**

Stand straight with good posture and take three deep breaths in and slowly out.

Imagine your feet growing roots, connecting deeply in the ground, reaching the centre of the earth. Feel that nurturing pulse and see her golden energy coming up the roots into your feet, up your spine, arms, and head, then cascading out from your crown and falling through your aura into the ground and back up your feet again.

Put your hands up to the sky and stretch up high like the tallest tree in the forest and smile. Imagine cupping your hands around the centre of the sun. Feel that powerful solar light pulsing down your hands, arms, head, and down your body, out of your feet, and back up through your aura to the sun and back down to you. Enjoy being totally earth and solar-powered.

You are feeling truly connected and safe.

Breathe in to the count of 7, hold it for 5, and release slowly for 7. Breathe normally.

Bring down your hands and place in prayer position.

If you haven't done so yet, please close your eyes, and release your neck so you can rest your chin down if you wish. Ensure your head is comfortable but your spine is stretched, chakras neatly stacked, meridians relaxed, knees slightly bent, and shoulders back. A good posture is important.

Now, stretch up your hands as you breathe in and open your palms to receive the wonders that are waiting for you. Breathe out as you bring your hands to your heart.

Do this three times.

Now, stretch up again, and bend slowly from your hips until your hands reach the floor, or your knees, however far you can bend safely, is fine. If you can reach the ground then place your hands onto the grass or the floor and hang there, allowing your spine to relax. Connect to the earth and repeat the words, out loud if possible:

I am grounded
I am rooted
I am nurtured
I am safe
I am pure femininity
I am me

Slide your hands up your legs as you unfurl your spine. Slowly stand up and continue sliding your hands up your body, over your face and head and back up to the sun. Stretch as tall as you can. Now, repeat these words whilst looking up:

I am powerful
I am solar
I am pure masculinity
I am real
I am me

Now, put your hands on your groin or bum and imagine a large bright red ruby lighting up your whole being. Say this:

I am safe

Breathe as you move your hands to your abdomen. Imagine a huge orange crystal, a carnelian, blessing you with its glow of joy. And say:

I am creative
I am sensual
I am joy

Take a deep breath and place your hands on your stomach. As you imagine this beautiful yellow crystal, a powerful, pulsing citrine radiating. Say:

I am powerful
I am me
I am only me and I am brilliantly enough

Take a deep breath and move your hands over your heart or cup your breasts. And imagine a beautiful green emerald nurturing you, as you say these words:

I am love
I am full of wonder

Now bring your hands up to your throat and imagine a deep blue sapphire pulsing as you say:

I am infinite
I am authentic

Bring your hands up to cup your eyes and then stroke your temples. Imagine a bright comforting purple amethyst, as you say:

I am highly intuitive
I have amazing vision

Then slide your hands up to the top of your head, form a crown with your fingers, imagining a gold sun disc in the centre of it, as you say:

I am connected
I am amazing

Place your hands down your sides and push on the earth with your feet to activate her nurturing connection further. Allow that feeling to come up your feet and settle in your pelvic area, from there, squeeze your pelvic muscles and imagine your truest energy going up your spine through all your chakras and spouting out of your crown, shooting up and then cascade down through your aura and back to the ground and then back up through your feet again, this is a continuous flow. It is a constant fountain of your own precious energy frequency.

As you feel this rush gushing up all your connected chakras, say to yourself:

I am orgasmic

Relax and gather your external energy:

Take a deep breath with the intention to call back all of you, the parts of you that have been left behind either in bed or during your last holiday, you don't need to know where. Just say as you click your fingers, or ring an imaginary bell:

I call back all of me, now.

And feel your energy coming back to you, filling you up and completing you as you state:

I am present
I am here and now
This is me

Then bow to your own majestic-ness. Acknowledge that today you are grounded in your truest essence, and you now attract similar wonderful energies.

You are fully aware of all in your life and all the opportunities aligning your way.

Smile as you feel this gratitude and affirm:

I am bliss
I am love
I am gratitude
I am presence
Thank you
I love my life

You have now set yourself up for the most gorgeous day possible. Whatever happens in your day, you can take a deep breath and reconnect to this flow. It is your birth-right to be this connected and happy.

This does not mean that challenging things won't happen. It means you can remain centred in your true being and not be put off balance by the chaos around you.

You navigate it well, looking for the positives in all situations and what the universe has to teach you and bless you with.

If you do this every day, you will increase the impact it has on your life.

Give yourself this gift every morning, just for you.

It will help brighten the day and be in the space to make better health choices.

If you wish to stay in this space longer, add some yoga movements before closing your ceremony, take more deep breaths, if you learn chi-kung or tantric breathing then incorporate some here.

You can add a longer gratitude section when you say thank you at the end.

Thank you for my life and all in it, including, and then list some of the people, things, possessions, money, miracles, work, situations, hobbies, neighbours, friends, family, animals, trees, books, everything you can think of that bring you joy.

Energy begets similar energy, and so if you spend time in gratitude, the universe will send you more things to be grateful for.

You can make this morning ritual as long or short as you like and it can differ every time. Just know whatever you do is enough and is working.

You can give yourself a 'power sentence' that connects with this energy field.

Repeat it in your head or out loud anytime during the day or night to help boost that frequency; this is a quick hack.

After you have done this meditation several times, find your own sentence that feels real to you and this will become your personal mantra.

Until you find your own, feel free to use this one as I have embedded it with this meditation energy and so it is powerful for this purpose:

I am here and I am me, so in gratitude, mote it be.

It can be shortened to, but with a similar impact:

I am presence.

Thank you for taking this precious time to clean your energy field and be fully present in the world: we need you here.

I wish you a wonderful and magical day.

## Meditation 4: Emergency Bladder Rescue

This is for when you have cystitis or the signs that one is coming.

I know you are in pain and frustrated and want to be left alone right now. So if you can take yourself somewhere dark, comfortable and quiet, where you can be alone with your rescue team and focus on your bladder, then do so, if not there is always the coat-on-head option. You got this.

This will help you to weather the storm and calm your bladder. You are not alone. Your rescue team is here.

Leave the anger, frustration and any victim energy outside the door. The more love and understanding you can bring right now, the more effective the rescue mission will be.

Lay down somewhere warm, safe, and quiet if possible. If you are unable to leave the toilet, then switch the light off and sit up straight placing your hands on your bladder.

Take a deep breath and state out loud your intention:

'This is a rescue mission to help soothe my bladder.'

Visualise going straight into your bladder, or taking your blue submarine there.

And remember the signalling system you agreed with your bladder, let that lead you to where you need to be.

Once there, have a look around, no judgement, no changing anything yet, just be present in the centre of the storm in your bladder. Whatever it is, is fine.

Remember your daily morning ritual, that energy field you have set up, and connect to that. In all the love and presence you can muster, say your power sentence mantra, or the following:

I am safe
I am love
I am presence

Be the grounded centre that your bladder needs. It is drowning and fighting for you, be appreciative of that and hold out your hands to it. The more love and gratitude you can gift it, the more powerful the medicine.

See yourself sitting or standing in the middle of the raging sea. You send out a beacon of pure love, understanding and forgiveness. On a loud tannoy, so that your entire bladder can hear, repeat these words as you send out blue healing light. Imagine you are a lighthouse with this light swirling, illuminating the entire cave and the ocean.

I am safe
I am me
I am only me and I am brilliantly enough

I understand

I am sorry

Please, forgive me

I love you

I love you

I love you

Thank you.

All is well and I am resetting, now.

Push a big golden button. Witness the scene reset itself, fireworks over the water raining down calming energies. It could be that all the chaos gravitates to the lighthouse and just vanishes, leaving clear blue skies and a calm sea.

Or a golden globe embracing the whole bladder radiating love. Be fully present now. This is probably the first time you are fully present during a cystitis attack. This is where you need to be, your presence will help heal you. Be the best *you* that you can bring and trust that you are enough.

When your bladder needs you the most, you are there, holding its hand. You provide the safe space it needs to fight any infection and release the inflammation. It can now let go of the anger, the storm, the germs, it is safe, for it is loved.

It is important to connect at an energy level and awareness with your bladder now, and then do what you can in the physical world afterwards.

In this state of presence, centred connection, make yourself and your bladder a promise that you will keep:

'Bladder, I do not leave you, I am here. I will do the necessary at the physical level too. I will drink at least 2 litres of clean water today, if not more, to flush away the germs and rinse your sore walls. I will drink some high-quality aloe vera, at least a large glass, to help soothe you and give you the physical nutrients needed to heal yourself. I will drink organic herbal teas that help. I will not eat any inflammatory foods or drinks or smoke. I will have good foods to help you. I will rest, and I will be mindful of putting myself first because I matter and I am worthy of a happy body.

Bladder, if there is anything else you need from me, tell me. I am listening.'

Then listen. Use your senses.

It may just need you to remain present longer so you can hold the safe space for it to sob and cry or shout. It may want to tell you stories and dark secrets that it has been hanging onto for you that it doesn't want anymore. Memories of abuse, unwanted intrusions, people taking the piss out of you, controlling you, belittling you, pissing you off, the school bully, when you lied about having cystitis to get off work…

Just listen.

That is OK, it is a blessing to release, you are ready to let those frequencies go, and leave your bladder for good. Do what you need to not judge or attach anger to these energies or memories, just let them pass as you remain centred and in gratitude for all because now, all is well.

When you feel ready, remind your bladder that you are always there. Leave a representative of you, in any form you feel, is right. It could be you in a nurse uniform, or a golden or blue lighthouse, like leaving a light on in the hall as your bladder sleeps.

And now open your eyes, take a deep breath and activate the physical emergency protocols:

Have a wee, gently.

Drink a large glass of high-quality aloe vera.

Drink 2 to 4 litres of water during the day and evening.

Drink organic herbal teas known to soothe bladders.

Do not wear underwear, or if you do, then only lose organic ones.

Have a warm shower or a bath, being mindful of products and water quality.

Have positive self-talk.

Watch something funny with a warm hot water bottle on your tummy or lower back.

Remember all will be OK soon, but right now, your bladder needs extra care, and so do you.

Well done on taking this massive step, it has helped more than you know.

## Meditation 5: Bladder Cancer Transformation

You and your bladder need a big hug; I'm sending one right now through the magic of this page. I understand from people I know with this condition, that cancer in the bladder is unbearable, and of course, it would encourage cystitis, as well as potential despair morally and emotionally. So, this is about allowing the fear and the despair to take a holiday whilst we increase hope and relief.

Please do all the meditations, not just this one, but if you have cancer, do this every day. Even if you don't feel as if it is doing anything, trust that at some level it is.

Note: I do not wish to belittle your pain or how serious cancer is. I also realise that cancer needs medical help and that some people may not, sadly, recover from it. But just for now, let us imagine that we can heal ourselves and that energy and the way we see things can make a difference, OK? Cool. Thanks. So let's get into it.

Please get comfortable; lying down would be preferable. Prepare your healing space. Light a white, orange or blue altar candle or use a fake candle for safety. Sage the room first. Massage some organic aromatherapy diluted oils on your tummy and lower back. Get naked or in lose pyjamas or under the duvet. And make sure you have put the ' do not disturb' sign up. This is *your* time.

Once you are comfortable, place your hands over your bladder and close your eyes.

Take a deep breath in and hold it for the count of three and release the breath slowly.

Do this 3 times.

Breathe in again and as you breathe out state:

I am safe.

I am present.

I am here and now.

Imagine the golden nurturing sap coming from the earth into your feet and bladder.

Now, imagine the white angelic light from the sky coming down into your crown and down your body into your bladder.

See the two powerful energies linking up and forming a circle of magic, engulfing the whole lower body area.

Take a deep breath and announce:

'This is a deep healing session. The power of Earth is nurturing me and the power of the Sky is healing me.

I am transforming. All is well.'

Then feel free to breathe as you wish, no longer any need to pay attention to your breathing rate.

See a swirling light that the Earth and Sky energies have formed and follow it to its centre.

The centre of this energy is in the middle of your bladder.

See yourself in the heart of it all. Take a look around.

I want you to really see the cancer. How does it show up? It could be green blobs on the walls. It could be craters, like bomb sites. It could be little creatures. It could be flowers. It could be just light or dark spots. It could be a fleet of Tai Fighters or Borg cubes. Whatever shows up is perfect. And it could be different each time, and that is OK too. And if nothing comes, that is fine, just acknowledge the cancer is there, and that it is listening.

The following message is now being transmitted:

'Hello, Cancer. It's me, your host. I know you are scared and confused. I've come to help you. You are not an intruder, you are not an infection or an invading army.

You are me.

Listen to me: I'm sorry. Please, forgive me. I love you. I thank you.

Oh, Opono Pono.

You are cells that have lost their way. You received the wrong information. You are working so hard and fast to reproduce yourself. I give you permission to stop.

Rest for a while. Let's hang out.'

It is important now to be as loving as possible. If you do see your cancer as something you consider evil, or invasive, perhaps right now you could change that image into something you love or care about. See cute animals, flowers or a tribe of giggling minions.

This is to change the energy frequency that you are sending your body.

Now, imagine gathering up the magic from the centre of the Earth and Sky energy. Create a large diamond from it.

See the magic swirl in this diamond. Now, in your mind, reach out to the back of your skull and pull out a draw. From here you will see a single cell. This is your truest blueprint. Your original cell containing all your DNA at the healthiest level.

Put this cell into the diamond and see it merge with the magic.

See a new original cell form in the draw and replace it in your skull, then forget it.

Pour love into this diamond.

Duplicate this diamond enough so that each of your cancer representatives gets one.

When you have them ready, speak to your faulty cells again:

'Dear cells, previously known as *Cancer*. I now delete your faulty instructions. I clear out the negative frequency.

And I gift you with this.'

Hand each one a diamond. Tell them:

'This is the purest cell of who we truly are. This contains the information you need to work properly. This will bring you back home.'

See them eat this diamond, or embrace it. Notice that swirling light surround them.

Watch as they each transform, from what they looked like, to a beautiful star-shaped cell, burning brightly and magically. They are happy.

They are transformed. No longer cancerous. They are happy cells. No longer confused, no longer working too hard or too fast.

Enjoy this transformation.

Stay in this space of healing, transformation, and gratitude for as long as you like.

With a grateful heart, it's time to let the cells get back to work, to their true purpose, in harmony with the rest of your healthy body.

State:

The cancer has gone.
I am healed.
I am whole.
My beautiful diamond DNA is empowering me.
My glowing star-shaped bladder cells are happy, possibly singing as they work.

My bladder is clear and strong.
All the cells in my bladder are now clear and original.

I am safe.
I am present.
I am positive and optimistic, for I know that all is well.

Take a deep breath and rub your tummy. Trace a love-heart on it.

Open your eyes and smile.

Well done. Really.

You have taken giant steps to relief, to potential recovery.

Do this every day.

It may be that after the first time you only see happy cells, and that is OK.

If that is the case then still hang out with them and boost them with the earth, sky, and your diamond cell magic, daily.

Make sure you gift yourself with this quality transformational time regularly.

Wishing you and your bladder a gorgeous day.

* * *

## Chapter 10 Keynotes

- Meditation is crucial to our well-being.

- Meditation doesn't need to take hours to be effective.

- Doing a daily morning ritual will help set up your best day, do this every day and it helps to set up a happy life.

- When you have cystitis of any type, do the emergency protocol, which includes the meditation I designed.

- Cancer is a negative word describing confused or rogue cells. Changing the name to something positive may help change its frequency.

- Stating an identity rather than a possession is stronger in affirmation. *I am love* is stronger than *I am loved*.

## Action! Interactive bit, it's your turn:

1. In your journal, write down your morning ritual, and start doing it.

2. Record or familiarise yourself with all the meditations again and do them, then record your experiences.

3. Write in your journal any comments or thoughts that come up during any meditation.

4. What is your power sentence?

So, we have enjoyed blissfully meditating together and are chilled out. Now let's explore taboos and social shackles that may be holding us back.

Let's tank it to Chapter 11.

# CHAPTER 11

# Breaking Taboos & Shedding Social Shackles

It's time to break taboos around women and liberate ourselves from the shackles of society.

What do I mean by that?

Great question.

A taboo is something, so a subject, a thought, a belief, an idea, an action, a rule or whatever, that we are told to suppress, to hide, to sweep under the carpet, something that one just doesn't talk about. It is considered rude, embarrassing, offensive, dirty, against the norm, frowned upon, judged, or just plain wrong.

It is also a belief that has been socially accepted, sometimes without question, or a cultural or traditional belief that, in my opinion, no longer serves us.

Breaking taboos means calling them out. Naming them, exploring them, understanding what they mean and how they affect us.

Then, if we decide we no longer wish to be a part of that taboo, we unlock the chain that binds us to it. We shed the shackle and walk away for good.

So, breaking a taboo is calling it to attention so we know what we are dealing with.

Liberating ourselves from its shackle is making a conscious decision that we are no longer tied down by that cultural/social/traditional belief.

We don't destroy the taboos themselves as we are not able to. They are powerful entities that have been around since man invented them, gathering power with each person who plugs into it.

All we can do is unplug ourselves and regain our part of the energy that powered it.

When enough people unshackle themselves from a particular taboo, it will dissolve. Ah, what a wonderful world that would be.

In this chapter, and indeed throughout this book, we are going to break several taboos, aimed mainly at women's health and the urinary tract.

This subject is vast and can be really intense, so I will write another book solely on breaking taboos, as this one is primarily about bladder health, but let's start the process and touch upon two relevant ones here. OK? Cool.

## Some Specific Taboos Affecting Women

### Taboo: as a woman, it is your duty to produce children.

This comes from when our species was low and in constant danger of starvation or being eaten by predators. A belief was born that women have to have children to help the race survive. This continued in Victorian times (UK) as the children mortality rate was high; we needed plenty of off-springs for some to make it to child-bearing adulthood.

Although this may have been a positive reason at the time, it is no longer useful.

This taboo is partly responsible for the now over-populated planet; we have a surplus of people and in the UK far too many habitats and countryside are being destroyed in order to build yet more housing to meet the ever-increasing demand of the population. Humankind is so rife that it is killing off other species.

This taboo is also partly responsible for the 'empty nest syndrome', when a woman feels bereft, lost and of no use once her children are grown up.

### Shedding the shackle:

Womanhood has *nothing* to do with motherhood.

We have enough people now to populate the Earth, even if all women of child-producing age decided not to get pregnant.

You are no more of a woman because you have children and you are no less of one.

A woman is a woman, complete without having to do anything else.

A mother is a woman choosing to adopt the role of being a mum.

Sometimes a woman will choose to be a mother, sometimes she won't, and that is OK, either way, she is still a woman.

I know women who are desperate to conceive, whose strong need to have their own biological children is all-encompassing. That is fine too; I understand the need to have someone to love unconditionally. Goddess knows I would not be without felines in my life. However, the pressure this creates can be devastating to a woman's health and her marriage. I suggest if you definitely want children and are not prepared or within the strict criteria to adopt, then be as kind to yourself and to your partner during the whole *trying to get pregnant* process, as the lighter you can keep your frequency, the better the chance of conceiving. There are lots of treatments that can help; one I strongly believe in is acupuncture. My acupuncturist (who treats me for other issues) is an expert in the field of fertility.

My point is that if you are able to conceive and chose not to or do have kids, or if you are struggling getting pregnant or not able at all, it does not affect your womanhood or femininity.

You are amazing. Children may be a welcome addition to your life, and you would not be without them once you have them, and yes, you would die for them, but they are not your whole reason to exist.

You were here and alive and *enough* before you had children.

You may choose to experience being a mother or a wife, but you are a woman regardless.

The woman *you* have been all through your life, and the *you* that existed before you were born and will continue to live on eternally, is *always* there, regardless of your human, social or parental circumstances.

Loosening the apron strings/flying the nest syndrome: once her children are grown up, a woman's practical, hands-on mothering duties may have slowed down or ceased, but she is still a complete woman.

Going back to work or staying at home once being a mother is up to you or your financial situation, but not up to society or taboos.

**Note**: if you are considering having children for negative (low-energy ) reasons, such as to get more benefits, free housing, to please a man, to feel validated as a woman, because it's what is expected of you from others or society, then consider not having children, as those reasons may eventually cause blockages in your body and dampen your field to keep you stuck in spiralling belief patterns.

I am unable to have children; something I don't often discuss, not because I'm ashamed or embarrassed, but because it doesn't define me or stop me living my life in any way. I'm grateful to be alive and make the most of finding out how I can manifest miracles and create life in different ways, and writing books is one of those.

That said I wasn't always OK and had to clear emotional blocks around it. I was also judged or treated differently because I chose not to have children when I could (due to lack of a decent man!), because I could no longer have children, because I didn't want to freeze my eggs or go through invasive procedures to try to get pregnant, because I didn't want to adopt, because I didn't go find a divorced man with children I could call my own... Bla, bla, bloody, bla.

I know women who were judged because they had children too young, too old, adopted even though they could conceive, delivery at home, in the hospital, got pregnant by sperm donor and raising the child alone, gay couples having children, breastfeeding in public, not breastfeeding, which schools to enrol their toddlers in...and the list is so bloody endless.

*Yawnsville! I'm so friggin underwhelmed by these taboos.*

I'm totally bored with women's taboos and varying society's expectations. Aren't you?

Some of the judgements and opinions, by the way, came from other women, mainly those with children. Can we not just agree to disagree and just be happy with what we have and our own choices, and respect others for standing by their decisions?

So ready, unshackle and walk away. We are free from this debilitating taboo.

Yippee!!!!!

**Taboo: you need to be ladylike. Women don't cuss. Women don't sweat, they shine. Women's poo smells like roses. Women don't fart. Women do sewing and cook. Women should have decorum. Women should cover-up. Women should not talk about their time of the month. Women are weak and hysterical. Women should...**

This started probably in the cave-age when there were clearly defined roles between men and women. Back then it was not insulting but true of the times, to some extent. The men were stronger build and had the instinct to fight and hunt. Women were smaller and they were the only ones who could bear children and therefore made a home. During those times life expectancy was much shorter and there was no medical or holistic help, so many women died in childbirth, and if they made it through, adults-only lived to about 30. That meant that being a mother was your whole life, and if you were not able to have children, your man and therefore the food-supply and protection, would leave you, so not having children made you somewhat more vulnerable.

This taboo grew as the man had power when cultures evolved. Money, industry, borders and politics were invented. Men were more aggressive as they evolved from hunting and were more suited to these positions and therefore the woman was still considered the weaker sex. They were still seen as needing protection. They were then considered as property. They were not deemed intelligent or worthy of much, certainly not the vote, or have any kind of say, even in pregnancy, as the pill was not invented yet, and when it was, women taking it were seen as dirty, cheap or turning against femininity. Women got pregnant if they wanted to or not, as a husband had rights and rape wasn't really an issue, especially between husband and wife.

Women were portrayed as trophies with their husbands showing off who had the best prize. Therefore women were taught to be proper, had elocution lesson to speak like a lady should walk as a lady should, act like a woman was expected to (according to men, mainly). She was dedicated to her man, her homemaking and to her beauty, always ensuring she looked good, wore the right clothes, said the right things, acted superbly and devoted to her man, or the pursuit of finding one.

It is only very recently that this has changed. Women only got the vote equal to men in 1928 in the UK, and in some parts of the world, this is *still* not the case. Suffragettes would turn in their grave knowing women are still treated as second-rate in some parts of the world. They probably despair that women in the UK have the vote and don't use it.

In some cases, we still, in 2019, don't have full equality in earning equal wages in the same job or have equal respect in certain industries.

### Shedding the shackle:

*Enough!*

*It ends here.*

*None* of the reasons or cultural beliefs that women are second rate, the weaker sex, need to land a man, be the best trophy, should cover-up, or don't have bodily functions, are valid anymore.

We no longer need to take a man's name in marriage, what's the point? We have our own names, right? We no longer need to be attached to an affluent man or marry into the right family for society image or financial reasons. We no longer need to be married. Women can be single all their life, and still, survive!

Names are important, they have power, and your name was yours since birth. It means something and it forms part of your aura and frequency, whether you like your name or not. By changing your name to fit into an outmoded cultural system, you change that part of your vibrancy; you cut away or at least dampen the part that resonated to your maiden name. Sometimes the effects won't be noticeable, sometimes they are.

This forms part of the reason why some women after being with the same partner for years, get married to them and then within a couple of years they are divorced. They are of course countless reasons contributing to divorce, but partly it is because a woman no longer feels like herself, too different after marriage, an identity crisis happens. Name-change is partly responsible for that. I say that as men don't often say that is a reason they want a divorce, but I hear it a lot in women.

I also noticed that divorced women who legally change their name back to their maiden name tend to find themselves again, it can be most empowering.

That said, I know when ridiculously in love, we want to take his name, it's exciting, different, you feel closer to him. And he will obviously still expect it, although that is no reason to do it: it's not up to him.

Would he be so willing to change his family name? Ah, absolutely not, what about equal rights?

I don't like people expecting others to do what they are not prepared to.

**Double standards have gone on long enough between men and women.**

So if you decide you want to change your name in marriage and that feels right and fair to you, then, obviously go ahead and enjoy the process, it's your right to choose.

I spent most of my Religious Education (R.E) lessons (yawn bloody yawn) practising my new signature when I was to marry my childhood sweetheart because at 16, 17 and 18 I knew he was the one. I finally nailed it when he dumped me.

Apparently, he didn't get the memo that we were a forever couple.

And I'm so glad that I didn't marry him or change my name for any of my exes, because they quite obviously were not forever, and did not merit me taking their identity/name. I'm rather proud and happy to have my own identity and name, thank you very much.

It is *beyond* proven now that women are equal to men in terms of intelligence, being smart in various ways, strength, maths, business, politics, finance and all of society's requirements. Equally, men can be awesome cooks, housekeepers and mannies.

Finally, it is time for women to stand up, stand tall and know that in darkness during all these aeons, she has found her light.

By being true to you, to what you stand for, to who you are with warts and all, you find strength. By accepting our body as it is right now, we empower ourselves to make changes, by leaving the past behind including all of its shackles behind, we strive forward with earnest momentum.

## Women's bodily functions are human- no more hiding or being coy:

Let it be known globally, loudly and proudly: women have human bodies.

We fart, burp, poo, pee, have facial hair, body hair, and sweat. During the menopause, we could beat any man at a sweating competition, and we can hold our own in a farting one too, anytime.

My hormonal moustache and rogue chin hairs gave me free passage into Mexico.

*Decorum?* Bollocks to that.

*Elocution lessons?* Piss off.

*Damsel in fucking distress?* Get a life.

How's that for ladylike? Oh, I should wash my mouth out with soap. Yeah, right.

Ladylike can go fuck itself along with the men that invented that taboo or still hang onto it, and that includes those women who still think it is OK to judge or slag off other women for their choices.

As a woman, if you choose to be ladylike, whatever that means to you, or take your husband's name, that's fine because you chose it, not chained to it subconsciously. It's just not my bag, but I won't judge you if it's yours.

Ladylike is not womanhood. Just like motherhood, it is a choice that a woman makes, it does not identify her as a woman.

Be who you are and know that you are brilliantly enough.

**You are now unshackled from this taboo.**

Boom (*Mike drop*).

Go forth freely into the world and illuminate – and fart, should you wish to.

## Linguistic Clues

Anything that blocks our emotional or mental *flow* will affect our body too.

So if someone is *wound-up* (wound up tightly stops the flow) they may end up with colon or urinary issues, as they are not allowing the flow.

If someone is so *uptight* that they have *a pole up their own arse*, it stops the flow of poo (emotional toxins) and any flexibility.

*Taking the piss* is not allowing it to flow where it is supposed to go and therefore linked to stopping urine flow freely at the physical level.

Being *so tight* in terms of stress, worry about money, and rigid in beliefs or body, inhibits the flow of money and everything, including our bodily functions of elimination such as pooing and peeing.

As we already know, we left clues in our languages to help us understand the bridge between metaphysical and physical.

*By now I'm guessing you are aware of your speech and how others talk as these linguistic interludes are eye-and-ear-opening, right?*

## Women's Health

As we have established that we too have a human body and that other than a few differences, male and female are almost the same biologically (we have a clitoris, they have a penis. We have a womb and ovaries, they have testicles, we both have breasts, facial and body hair) therefore it is totally acceptable and natural to discuss any of our body parts or problems.

All parts of the body are equal and none are shaming, embarrassing, funny, or taboo.

This book is primarily about bladder and precious holes, however following the protocols will have a positive effect on your whole body, especially your vulva, perineum, womb and colon, because treating all of your precious holes will enhance the areas that they lead to as well.

Following the dietary recommendations may also improve all of the digestive tract, energy levels and your skin.

Using the recommended supplements and personal care products could help other systems too.

By ensuring you do not get thrush in the bladder, you also avoid thrush in the vagina, anus and bowels.

If you follow the sexual protocols you should avoid thrush or itchy vulva after sex too.

**Note:** pregnancy and sexually transmitted diseases are only avoided by not having sex at all, or by using a condom, although condoms are not 100% effective.

So by reading this book and implementing the suggestions within it, you are essentially helping all of your systems. The entire body will benefit from treating your bladder right. By dealing with one inflammation issue properly, we essentially treat them all.

**So to be clear:**

If you have issues with your womb, vagina, clitoris, bladder, urethra, colon, anus, ovaries, fallopian tubes, pubes, facial hair, breasts, belly-button or *any* body parts, or suffer with menopause, period pain, constipation, toilet problems, cystitis, fertility issues, incontinence or dry precious holes, it just means you are a woman and need some help: *speak out.*

There is no shame in treating yourself right at all levels and stating proudly that your health matters.

If other people have a problem with you speaking out or asking for what you need, it really is *their* problem. There is no shame in any part of the human body, and none of it should be a taboo.

I invite you now to get naked, sit on the floor and spread your legs. Either sit in front of a mirror or use a hand-held mirror and look at your bits. Explore, see what you look like down below. It is all part of *your* body: love it.

\* \* \*

Gone are the days, thank goodness, when women being all coy and pathetic about things is normal. Luckily, girls no longer need to hide in huts to bleed, considered weak or dirty, are called whores for wanting sex, or evil for having sex outside of marriage, or considered as property. Periods, hormone changes, facial hair, developing boobs and curvy hips, menopause, sweating, peeing, and pooing are just part of having a female body. They are *normal.*

What is *not* normal about being a woman: being beaten, in the past husbands could hit their wives with a stick no thicker than their thumbs (where the saying *the rule of thumb* comes from), working the same job as men but for less pay, not allowed to vote, not allowed an opinion, when illness or being outspoken was put down to women's hysteria and weakness.

Voting, equal pay, respect, and choices should now be a part of human society, so men and women are treated the same. If you live in a country where this is not yet the case, then hopefully you will soon. It's 2019 people, time to wake the fuck up. Women are amazing and life-giving, it's time all men, governments and religions realise that.

Remember where we all (men and women) came from: an egg, down a fallopian tube, then a male orgasm impregnating the egg, then the womb and finally entered the world via the vagina. It is the female body that gave you life, carried you and nurtured you. By disrespecting or belittling any girl or woman, you are essentially insulting yourself and all human life.

When you feel down just remember that *you* won the race and up to 499,000 others failed. Yes, there can be up to ½ billion sperm per ejaculation. Only one made it: you.

It had to make it when the right and fertile egg (also you) was ready and willing to receive. It had to happen when all the circumstances were favourable to gestation. Your mother had to be in the best state to carry you to term and give life to you. Then you had to survive in this modern society amongst all the bullshit, heartache and limiting beliefs, to be where you are today.

**You, my Darling, are a winner**. Just for being you, right as you are now, you have conquered so much, celebrate that. I am.

For those women who still feel abandoned, abused or who are forced to hide their femininity by religion, governments, culture or under the influence of a control freak, remember that one thing that can never be taken away from us is our thoughts. You have the choice of what to think and feel. It's easier said than done, but I hope you can take strength from other women around the world.

It's time women stood strong together. No longer the second rate, no longer under the rule of men, religion or taboos.

Imagine if all women loved each other, respected each other and stood together.

Let's energetically do that now.

*Come on, stand up and really visualise.*

See yourself as a part of a strong beautiful world-changing energy ring around the planet. Hold out your hands and energetically connect with a woman on each side and see them do the same, feel the energy of the circle.

I don't like labels or boxes. If anyone tries to shove me in one, and they have throughout my life, I rebel and break free, that's just who I am: a taboo-breaking rebel, but if I'm left alone to be *me*, then I have no need to rebel.

I'm not a rebel without a cause, but I do insist on living my life my way, it took me over four decades to realise that was the point.

So a woman is a woman. It doesn't matter what roles she adopts or what she looks like: skin colour, race, feminist, neutral, financial situation, single, married, lesbian, heterosexual, bi-sexual, everything-sexual, monogamous, orgy-sexual, sleeps around, celibate, virgin, tall, short, fat, thin, passionate, quiet, introvert, extrovert, swears, well-spoken, tattooed, waxes, fully-bushed, educated, home-schooled, working, career-minded, mother, not a mother, fertile, barren, healthy, suffering from women's issues, depressed or joyful.

A woman is a woman.

**To be fair, a man is a man, the same 'rules' apply. I'm about harmony.**

**Dude, I do love you too.**

So I would like to point out that this book is not about bashing men or blaming others for our situations. I was brought up in a family of many loving and amazing men. I also fell in love with some really shitty men.

Lucky in family, unlucky with lovers. One of my best friends is a man. Men are bloody brilliant too in their own way on their own path.

**So I'm not a feminist (if we want to use a label), I believe in people.**

Gender, age or religion play no part.

If you are a kind-hearted man, I'm gonna like ya.

If you are a kind-hearted woman, I'm gonna like ya.

If you are any kind of fauna, flora or gem, I adore you unconditionally.

If you are a cat, instant lurve and ooooh I will love you forever.

If you are a two-timing lying arsehole shit-bag of a man, I'm probably gonna fall for ya, dammit! I'm working on that no longer being a repeated lesson for me.

**So just to sum up: I love women. We are bloody brilliant, all of us.**

I'm not a lesbian but I respect and admire femininity and womanhood.

I'm part of a fantastic sisterhood that keeps getting stronger. There is nothing sexier and more inspiring than witnessing a woman lose the layers of crap and unfurl into her true self, her shiny beautiful unique self, and then bring that light to the world, encouraging others to do the same.

How about we create a world where we respect humans, no longer defining what a man or woman should be?

If a man is gay and decides to raise a family with his husband, and he is happy, that is his right, just as a man being with a woman and having a family, or a man deciding to be single: any man following his heart can't go wrong.

Any woman following her heart can't go wrong. It may not be easy, I'm sure it won't be, but living your true life is surely the only way during the short time on this glorious planet. Right?

However you form a family, it's a family. Love knows no gender nor genetic boundaries: love is love.

So I'm not a man-basher and I'm not saying women are better than men or that we are the superior sex. We have had to overcome so much shit put on us by men over the centuries, that I do have a penchant for us. Go, women! Rise, be free…

We are not the weaker sex or lesser than men. Women are finally able to rise and stand proud, showing the way for equal humanity. And I love that.

So before I gush too much: I love you.

* * *

Breaking taboos increases our awareness of what we are involved with, of what is sucking our energy.

Unshackling ourselves empowers our ability to choose and live in our own way.

So, breaking taboos and liberating ourselves from shackles means we gain back a lot of energy that we can use to charge up our own lives and health.

It empowers us to make our own decisions and reminds us that we are enough, just as we are. You then become a pioneer, as we can enhance our health and life by breaking free from taboos, then others may want to do the same.

Changing the world starts with you.

Just as taboos are negative, there are positive morphic fields too and plugging into those can enhance your energy and support you. We explored that in the Community Protocols earlier.

Whatever is happening in your reality, just know that you are supported. You are part of a global feminine love-circle of power: tap into it.

## Chapter 11 Keynotes

- Women's health issues are not taboo, shameful, funny or secret. Speak out.

- Breaking taboos means calling them out so we can deal with them.

- Unshackling ourselves gives us back our own power and energy.

- Taboos are negative thought-forms.

- There are positive energy fields too. The movement of *Piss to Bliss* is one.

- You are part of a global feminine power energy circle, so embrace it.

- Women are just bloody brilliant.

## Action! Interactive bit, it's your turn:

1. What have you read in this chapter that has enlightened you?

2. Write down the taboos that you are breaking and notice how you change as a result over the coming months.

3. Have you ever felt put down as a woman or unfairly treated?

4. What actions can you put in place so that you no longer allow unfairness or abuse in your life, either from others or from yourself?

5. Have you suffered from any women's health issues and not spoke out because you were too embarrassed or ashamed? Do you feel

more confident speaking out now? If not, notice how you may do as a result of reading this book.

6. Have you looked at your bits in the mirror yet? Had a good gander?

So, we have broken a few taboos around women's health and expectations and unshackled ourselves: welcome back to our long-lost energy!

It's time now to review those all-important protocols.

Come on, let's put the *pedal to the metal* because chapter 12 awaits…

# Chapter 12

# Protocols Summary/
# The A-Team Has Your Back

**The A-Team** reminds us that we all like it when a plan comes together.

So this is a summary, pulling the protocols together. It's in your hands now.

The A-Team way would be to tick all the 'good' boxes on a regular basis and never introducing any from the trigger team. This is ideally your aim.

So, start adopting one protocol at a time until they become second nature. Your bladder health will increase with each step.

It may be that you do the full A-Team for a set time, such as 8 weeks, to really clear your bladder. Then, reintroduce some things from the trigger list that you still want in your life. This could be an occasional blow-out meal; a night out getting pissed; the crazy off-the-cuff sex with someone with no sexual protocol; swimming in Jacuzzi and pools; smoking; staying up for days without sleep; not drinking enough water, or wearing thongs on occasion. Whatever your poison really.

Once you have reset, you can allow these things back into your life providing you take counter-measures and listen to your body for signals.

It is going to be trial and error as we are all different. We are all going to have different fulcrums, different balancing points. Keep a journal to correlate breaking protocols with symptoms.

The gold is in the details, read the full protocol chapter again and let it sink in.

No really, go on, I'll wait here and listen to our road-trip soundtrack.

Ah, you're back. Coolio. Let's continue our journey.

This chapter is useful as a quick glance.

You can write these out in your journal, or photocopy it and pin it up on your wall, in your diary, or put it in your handbag. Live with it until it becomes second nature.

Ready, let's dive in:

1. **Toilet Protocols**

   - Ensure a clean toilet

   - Use plain cotton loo roll

   - Place loo roll in the bowl to avoid splash-back

   - Wipe front to bottom only

   - Do not hang on to wee or poo, go to the loo as soon as you know

   - Relax and fully empty your bladder and bowels

   - Do not rush or push too hard

   - Use a 'Squatty Potty' when possible

- Rinse after each poo

- Wash hands thoroughly

2. **Daily Hygiene Protocols**

- Wash the body twice daily with appropriate products

- Use a special shower-head

- Ensure clean and safe water to cleanse with

- Use safe products and rinse really well

- Brush under your nails

- Wash hands properly after using the toilet

- Remember all the germs that your hands touch, so clean them often

- Brush teeth twice a day with an appropriate toothpaste

- Ensure your sexual partner is hygienic too

- Keep your flaps clean!

3. **Products Protocols**

- Remember everything you touch or use will affect your health

- Use animal-friendly and ethical products to ensure high energy frequency

- Beware of marketing ploys and brain-washing buzz-words

- Make your own truly natural and safe products

- Buy a trusted brand

4. **Sexual Protocols**

- Anything touching your precious holes may affect your bladder

- Vulva skin ( *your flaps*) are sensitive so beware of chaffing, irritants, nasty products, and germs

- Wax off pubes, trim beards, and avoid body hair chaffing sensitive skin

- Sex, even if clean, will cause some trauma to your pelvic area and bladder

- Avoid transference of all nasties: germs, bacteria, pubes, sweat, saliva, poo, pee, dirt, dead skin cells, food particles, E-coli, candida, fungi, either from you, your partner or your toys

- Do not use food or unsafe products for sex

- Sexual cystitis can happen even if there is no bacterium present

- Drink water before and after sex

- Have a pee straight after sex, gently

- Wash properly before and after sex; both partners

- Wash all sexual toys properly before and after use

- Use skin-friendly lubrication, if needed

- Avoid anal sex or ensure proper lubrication and washing before and after

- Ensure clean mouth and preferably no beards for oral sex

- In emergency situations, where no washing is available, use your mouth to suck your partner's fingers and penis before penetration: damage limitation

- Be brave and have the talk. Discuss with your partner what you like and don't like and be prepared to refuse sex if they are not going to respect your levels of hygiene or your stance on demanding respect

- Breathe deeply and don't hold your breath

- Be fully present in the moment

- Send a safe signal to the bladder that bashing is coming but so are endorphins and that all is well

- Do not cross over from the anus to the vagina without changing condom, or washing first

- Do not use flavoured condoms as they can burn your bits

- After sex make sure you pee, wash and drink water and aloe vera if possible. Place your hands on your bladder and send safe, comforting vibes

- Positive thinking will help break any negative belief patterns associated with sex or new partners and you getting cystitis or thrush. Break the belief pattern

- If sex is not consenting, then do what you can to avoid it

- Speak out and get help to clear sexual abuse, past or current

- Avoid sex if you or your partner are angry or have negative vibes. You are not an emotional punching-bag. Remember whatever energy or mood enters you, will affect you

- Be choosy about who you have sex with, remember their energy will linger in you for a potentially long time

5. **Food Hygiene Protocols**

- Everything you eat, drink, inhale or touch will affect your body

- Remember, being too nice is not good for you, speak out if food is bad

- The primary role of food is for fuel, to help your body function

- These are irritants and non-foods: gluten, dairy, sugars, sweeteners, chemicals, over-manufactured, junk, trans-fats, alcohol

- Ensure clean kitchen surfaces, inside the fridge, shelves, larders, cooking tops, ovens, floors, utensils

- Wash your hands before preparing food

- Use clean cutlery and serving dishes

- Rinse off properly after washing up, commercial washing up liquids can be irritating and carcinogenic

- Designated shelves for raw meat and other foods in the fridge

- Re-wash hands after touching raw meat and change utensils before preparing other foods

- Dine at restaurants with food hygiene certifications and good reputations

- Food is fuel, it is not part of sex so avoid rubbing it on your bits

- Avoid biting your nails

6. **Clothing Protocols**

- Avoid nasty materials: petrol, plastics, glues, chemicals, toxic dyes, and raw materials grown with pesticides

- Choose natural fabrics made from organic cotton, hemp, linen, bamboo, wool

- Beware of negative energy frequency; avoid buying clothes that are imbued with animal, human, or environmental abuse

- Avoid knickers wherever possible, go commando

- Avoid tight clothing around your vagina: trousers, leggings, tight knickers

- When knickers are necessary, so when wearing trousers to avoid chaffing, choose big, loose-gusseted, organic ones made from a natural material

- Do not wear thongs, strings, frilly lacy knickers. Ditch the cheese-slicers!

- Do not wear clothes that make you sweat or overheat down below

- Shower, dry, and change into dry clothes after exercising, or getting wet, do not sit in damp clothing

- Comfortable shoes or barefoot will help keep good posture

7. **Nutritional Protocols**

- Cut-back, avoid or better still, eliminate altogether the following:
    - Gluten
    - Corn/Maize
    - Dairy
    - Sugars, organic fruit in season is OK or raw honey on occasion
    - Fizzy drinks
    - Sweeteners
    - Alcohol
    - Cigarettes/tobacco
    - Pesticides/fungicides/chemicals/GMO
    - Caffeine and chocolate

- What to eat in abundance and mindfully:
    - Organic fruit and vegetables
    - Organic healthy oils such as olive, coconut, avocado, walnut
    - Wild-caught fish and seafood, not farmed
    - Wild meat if possible, if not then grass-fed and grass-finished, or grass-reared organic, free-range meat.

- We don't need much animal protein. Too much may affect the kidneys

- Beware of the energy of the meat you are eating, any abuse, force-feeding, or misery will be imbued in its flesh and so, then into you

- You are what you eat, and what your food ate, and how your food was treated

- Paying for cheap food that has been neglected or laden with chemicals is tapping into the energy of abuse, anger, sadness, grief, inauthenticity, going against nature and humanity and could have a negative impact on your health

- Quality is key: you get what you pay for

- Food is fuel, choose the good stuff that your body truly needs

- Beware of governments, the food industry, marketers and lobbyers, selling tactics. Who is profiting from your food choices and what impact does that have on your health and the planet?

- Encourage food combining, so not mixing proteins and carbohydrates in the same meal, e.g. no meat, tofu or pulses with potatoes, bread, rice …

- Increase anti-inflammatory and good-gut forming organic foods:
  - Lemon
  - Apple Cider Vinegar (organic with the mother)
  - Celery
  - Garlic
  - Onions
  - Ginger
  - Turmeric
  - Cinnamon
  - Raw organic extra virgin coconut, premium olive oil, walnut oil
  - Herbs
  - Organic herbal teas such as chamomile, mint, nettle, hibiscus, rosehip
  - Aloe Vera, the best quality as possible
  - Green vegetables, a wide variety, explore!

- Some fruit, but due to its nature, it needs to be eaten on an empty stomach so it passes through quickly, and seasonally is best
- Spring or mineral water, sadly most come in plastic bottles but it is still preferable to tap water unless properly filtered
- Red Tea

## 8. Hydration Protocols

- All drinks to be either room temperature or warm

- Avoid cold or icy drinks

- Warm water with lemon or ginger in the morning

- Sip 1.5 to 5 litres water during the day depending on your weight and situation

- More water if exercising, having sex, fever, run-down, dehydrated, hot day, on holiday in the sun, in air conditioning, travelling, or in aeroplanes

- Include high water-content food in your diet

- Avoid alcohol, caffeine, black teas, too many green teas, fruit juice or squash

- Drink naturally caffeine-free organic herbal teas

- Keep skin hydrated with dry skin brushing and massaging in organic coconut oil or other appropriate moisturisers

## 9. Stress Protocols

- Do the morning ritual meditation daily

- Do mindful deep breathing exercises during the day and before bed

- Identify your biggest stress factors and take action to reduce them

- Make relaxing time part of your habitual life: allow the stress to evaporate often so it doesn't build up and explode

- Try regular activities or treatments to help keep stress at bay: snogging, yoga, tai-chi, swimming, dancing, singing, cinema, theatre, fun community gatherings, stretching, painting, writing, reading, cooking, napping, meditating, reiki, retreats, counselling, massages, spa days, hugging animals...

- Have quality time with your pets or consider getting a pet from a shelter if you don't have one already and make 2 lives happier

- Have those difficult conversations, do not bottle stuff up

- Take long baths with organic essential oils or salt

- Consider counselling or life coaching if you are struggling

## 10. Clear Space Protocols

- Remember 'as within, so without'

- Energy begets similar energy

- Declutter at all levels:
  - **Without**: your environment, words, music, house, office, phone, car, clothes, possessions, air, surroundings, and your actions
  - **Within**: your thoughts, beliefs, lies, attitudes, grudges, self-talk, nutrition, smoking, drinking

- **Social**: your work, friends, colleagues, social networks, social media, emails, books, computer games, the news, media, piss-takers, bullies, hobbies

## 11. Metaphysical Protocols

- Crystals: use relevant crystals like carnelian, agate, onyx, to meditate, massage your tummy and lower back, put in your bath, have crystal reiki healing

- Chakras: the root, red, located at feet/legs and groin area. The sacral, orange, located in the lower abdomen. Massage or meditate on these areas and send loving energy to ensure they are clear and strong

- Colours: red, orange, brown, black and blue. Colour therapy, wearing these colours, bed linen or meditating with them in mind

- Elements of Water & Fire: water, for waterworks and emotional healing. Water is the main element of urine and the bladder is a water-bag. The sacral chakra is about creativity and joy and so fire is the element of creation and passion

- Essential Oils: ylang-ylang, clary sage, pumpkin seed, lavender, bergamot.

- Herbs: goldenseal, bearberry leaf, Pau d'arco bark, nettle, chamomile. Not cranberry

- Holistic treatments:
  - Regular massages
  - Acupuncture

- Reiki, crystal reiki and any hands-on-healing you trust, including remote healing from therapists afar, or even prayers
- Applying a hot water bottle or diluted oils on your tummy or lower back
- Drinking plenty of water and eating healthy foods

- **Stored Energies Protocols**

- Everything is related, everything matters and energy begets similar energy

- Physical level: the body, the environment, this planet

- Mental level: thoughts, belief systems, dreams, memories, lies

- Emotional level: emotions, feelings, memories, blocked energies

- Spiritual level: faith, deep rooted-beliefs about existence, religions, past-life memories & influences

- The main energies linked with the bladder are:
  - Frustration
  - Irritation
  - Anger
  - Piss-offness
  - Piss-takers. Abusers. Controllers. Narcissists, tabooers
  - Fear/Terror
  - Sexual abuse, rape, not saying no when you want to
  - Bed-wetting
  - Bullying
  - Piss-taking, making a joke out of you, negative sarcasm
  - Any emotional impact that shook you
  - Deep dark secrets, taboos or memories unleashed

- Self-loathing
- Being too nice/doormat
- Being in denial/sweeping stuff under the carpet
- Disconnection to self and body
- Alcoholism
- Heavy smoking
- Poverty Belief

## 12. Medical Protocols

- Cystitis is a big deal, get examined medically to rule out other issues

- Antibiotics are required to help combat bacterial infection cystitis/UTI

- If your doctor or urologist is useless or condescending, find a better one

- Medically trained people are often not experts on bladders or your body

- Build a team of professionals to help you with your bladder health at all levels and remember that YOU are in the driver's seat

## 13. Posture Protocols

- A good posture helps keep our organs, muscles and chakras well-stacked

- Apply good posture when sitting, standing, lying, bending or lifting

- Take deep cleansing breaths and breathe deeply

- Our core muscles and pelvic muscles help to keep our bladder in place

- Avoid high-heels

## 14. Exercise Protocols

- Move a lot during the day

- There is no need for gyms or long workouts

- Engage core strength when exercising or lifting weights

- Check with your medical team if you have a fallen bladder or IC before doing *any* exercise

## 15. Environmental Protocols

- Ensure good footwear and aids for walking in dangerous conditions

- Consider avoiding dangerous activities or situations

- Take measures to reduce chronic irritants

- Brace yourself before walking down any stairs or doing potentially dangerous activities and keep a strong core

## 16. Community Protocols

- Who you spend time with will affect your health: **monkey see-monkey do**

- **Welcome to our jungle**, join our Facebook group 'The Happy Bladder Tribe'

- Surround yourself with people and activities that make you feel good

- It is important to get advice from those who have conquered their nemesis

* * *

Now you are familiar with the protocols again, use the following trigger checklist when you next get ANY type of cystitis or a bladder problem.

It will help you analyse why you got it. Knowledge is power.

It could be a mixture of these or just one.

Remember not all of these will lead to a UTI, some may just be a trigger for a mild cystitis bout.

This extensive list is a combination of potential triggers to ALL the 25 types.

It is important to have analysed which type you had to help link the appropriate triggers.

I haven't put the triggers in order of types, that is up to you to work out, **that way it keeps you involved in this conversation**, and the more you are active here, the deeper the information will sink in. Go for it.

## Potential Trigger List (for all types of cystitis)

So ask yourself in the last three days did I experience any of the following?

- Got dehydrated

- Dirty toilet water splashed back

- Wiped from back to front (bottom to vagina and urethra)

- Sat too long on the toilet after pooing

- Rushed or over-pushed my pee or poo

- Had diarrhoea

- Held on too long to my wee or poo

- Used damp, scented or tracing paper loo roll

- Had vaginal or anal thrush

- Sat in damp clothing

- Got too cold or walked barefoot on cold tiles

- Drank icy drinks or too much ice-cream

- Didn't wash or change after exercising/sweating

- Bathed in questionable water, especially if abroad

- Been in swimming pools or Jacuzzis

- Used irritating products, fem-washes, or wipes

- Had a bath with too many oils, bubble bath or questionable products

- Changed my cleaning products or laundry detergent

- Had 'dirty' sex

- Masturbated with dirty fingers

- Did not go to the toilet after sex

- Did not wash after sex

- Has sex with a new partner

- Used flavoured condoms

- Had anal sex

- Had oral sex with a bearded or unhygienic partner

- Let my pubes get too long

- Been raped

- Said yes to sex when I didn't want to

- Been too nice

- Been really pissed off

- Been bullied or abused in any way

- Left tampon or sanitary towel in too long

- Used food or cheap lubricants for sex

- Came into contact with someone with a virus

- Had too much sugar, gluten, dairy or other inflammatory foods

- Got drunk or had too much alcohol

- Had too much coffee, chocolate or green tea (caffeine)

- Ate curry or chilli, something overly spicy

- Consumed contaminated food or drink

- Bit your nails or sucked dirty fingers

- Wore toxic/man-made fibre clothes or new jogging/yoga pants

- Wore tight knickers or trousers

- Wore thongs or G-strings

- Invested in abusive negative energy food, drink, clothing, products

- Had chemicals, pesticides, GM, nasties or sweeteners

- Been smoking or passive smoking too much

- Wore high-heels for too long

- Had any kind of trauma to the spine or nerves

- Started new medication with potential side-effects

- Been on a jerky rollercoaster, waterslides did contact sports

- Had trauma to the lower abdomen

- Been punched or abused in that region

- Had trauma to the coccyx area

- Had trauma to my precious holes or flaps

- Got my flaps dirty!

- Been overly stressed

- Had a shock

- Been terrified, fearful, been fretting or anxious

- Keeping a secret that is eating me up

- Covering something up

- Bottling something up

- Being inauthentic in any way

- Going against myself or my principles

- Depressed

- Feel like I am living a lie or someone else's life

- Menopausal

- Recently (in last 4 months) came off HRT

- Living in clutter

- Disruption such as moving house, divorce, changing jobs

- Rundown, feverish, been ill

- Had antibiotics

- Gone over your fulcrum tolerances

- Got really irritated or frustrated

- Travelled, especially in an aeroplane

- Sat in a strange or uncomfortable posture for too long

- Had a fall

- Used cystitis as an excuse to get out of something

- Had cranberry juice

- Had too much fruit, sugar or sweeteners

- Bad self-talk/berated myself

- Told myself I will get cystitis because… (self-fulfilling prophecy)

- Worried about money

- Had a medical procedure, cystoscopy, colposcopy, smear-test or numbing gel

- Had a coughing virus and coughed too long and too hard

- Sneezing too much or too powerfully

- Hanging around with questionable people

- Kidney infection or cancer

- Other bladder issues such as stones, ulcers, cancer, fallen, leucoplakia

- Had any urinary incontinence

- Used a catheter

- Diabetes

- Fibromyalgia

- Chronic Fatigue

- Dementia

- Exhaustion/lack of good sleep

- Pregnancy

- Miscarriage

- Given birth

- Made any recent changes to my lifestyle

- Been dieting or detoxing (trapped toxins will have to be released and so may cause discomfort as they pass.)

- Been releasing blocked emotions related to the bladder? (hence emotional detoxing as the pain that was trapped may be felt as it passes)

- Anything else you can think of? Remember cystitis and any pain is a signal from your body that something is wrong, or that you are detoxing. Be present within your body and ask

\* \* \*

## What a day on the anti-candida regime may look like. Adjust the schedule to suit.

If you are unsure of taking supplements for any reason, it is imperative that you check with your medical practitioner and always read dosages and labels for all vitamins, supplements and medications.

Sugar and carbohydrates feed candida so we avoid them. This makes this diet food-combining by nature, which is a good practice to get into. When you do introduce sugars or carbohydrates again, choose the healthiest ones (fruit, rice, sweet potato) and do not have them in the same meal as proteins (meat, fish, nuts, eggs, legumes).

**Note:** all food organic. All water and herbal teas and soups made with mineral water.

7 am

Wake up. Wee. Brush teeth using suitable toothpaste. Clean your tongue (with the back of your toothbrush if it has ridges, or with a clean tongue scraper).

Dry skin brushing with a vegan natural bristle body brush.

7.15

Drink/down a pint of warm water with the juice of an organic lemon (half made from water from the room temperature mineral bottle, the other half from mineral water boiled in the kettle)

7.20

Poo. Shower, (hot/cold/hot/cold) and finish with a cold shower for 2 minutes and pat dry with an organic cotton towel.

With love massage oil or cream all over your body, face and hands and whilst looking in the mirror with appreciation. Wear organic cotton or bamboo clothing or pyjamas.

8.00

Drink 100mls of high-quality aloe vera gel drink.

Take supplements that require an empty stomach.

8.10

Go outside. Take 8 deep breaths. Do yogic, tantric or chi-kung breathing exercises. Morning ritual meditation. Yoga stretches. State your power sentences and what you are grateful for. Thank the Earth for your amazing body.

9.00

Drink a large organic home-made green smoothie with one or two cloves raw garlic. Ensure to chew the smoothie first to start the digestion with the saliva. Drink slowly.

Have supplements that need to be taken with food. And S. Boulardii & probiotics.

9.30
Start cleaning your house. Drink herbal tea as you go along. Remember as within so without. Pick a room per day and declutter, be ruthless, chuck out all unwanted house-guests and parasites, at all levels. Down a pint of mineral water at room temperature. Go to the toilet whenever you need to and follow all protocols.
Clean the tidied room with natural products.

Noon
Drink a glass of warm water with 2 tablespoons of organic apple cider vinegar.
Lunch: fresh mixed lettuce leaves, spinach leaves, cucumber, onion, avocado, extra virgin organic olive oil, mixed seeds, raw garlic, wild salmon steak.
Eat mindfully, presently. Take Vitamin B supplements and iron with a hot lemon after food, even if you had them already.
Wash up. Tidy kitchen.

2 pm
Go for a gentle walk and breathe deeply. Think only happy thoughts. If need be then repeated your power sentence continuously. Drink water as you walk.

3 pm
Large hot water with freshly cut ginger and cinnamon and turmeric.
Stretching exercises, or holistic treatment such as acupuncture or massage.

4 pm
100 MLS high-quality aloe vera gel drink.

4.15 pm

Finish cleaning the room you decluttered earlier on. Can you get rid of anything else? Take note of any feelings, memories, or related stories whilst clearing out. Refill your cup with hot water – it should still have the ginger in it. Ensure by now you have had at least 2 litres of mineral water, preferably more than 3 litres, not including the smoothie or herbal teas.

6.15 pm

Dinner: high energy organic properly raised chicken or turkey (roasted or shallowed fried in coconut oil) with cooked green vegetables, drizzled with avocado or olive oil. Home-made green vegetable soup with pink Himalayan salt.

Any supplements requiring food. More probiotics.

7.30 pm

Tidy kitchen.

7.45 pm

Watch a funny movie or read an uplifting or educational book. Drink more healthy fluids.

9.30 pm

Have a warm bath with Epsom salts or Himalayan pink salt (at least 500grs, yes that's right ½ kilo or even a kilo) Soak for 45 minutes. Enjoy, relax, let the stories go. Rinse in the shower afterwards and pat dry. Lovingly lather your body in aloe vera cream or coconut oil.

10 pm

Drink warm coconut or homemade almond milk with turmeric and cinnamon.

Take your Omega 3, H.A and any other oil supplements. Brush your teeth.

10.15 pm

State three reasons why you are grateful to be alive. Rub your tummy with a magnet with the intention of healing. Drink 100mls high-quality aloe vera.

Go to bed with some crystals, including rose quartz. Sleep. When you wake up for a pee, ensure to replenish the fluids by drinking more water, even during the night.

* * *

## Chapter 12 Keynotes

- There are 16 major protocols that form your **Bladder A-Team**.

- There are many potential triggers that can cause bladder issues.

- What an anti-candida day could look like.

- Repetition is key to allow the protocols to really sink in.

## Action! Interactive bit, it's your turn:

1. Make notes in your journal of the protocols that stood out to you.

2. Photocopy or handwrite the protocols list and familiarise yourself.

3. Understand and make a list of any triggers to avoid.

4. Do the anti-candida diet for 8 weeks and record it in your journal.

5. Find your fulcrum and design your healthiest lifestyle.

6. Be present in your body during any pain and ask what the message is. Analyse past cystitis bouts to ensure you get all the information.

We have revisited the all-important protocols and triggers.

*This plan has come together!*

I trust that you are well informed as we move on to the last chapter.

Come on: we are still holding hands.

# CHAPTER 13

# Time to Say Goodbye

Wooooooooooooo, what an adventure! We are back home, saying ta-ta.

So here we are, this is where I wish you super-well on your continuous journey.

My job here is done, and yours is truly beginning.

My aspirations for this book was to help you gain as much knowledge as possible about your bladder and precious holes, at all levels. To introduce you to basic metaphysics and change your perspective so that your nemesis becomes your best friend. It was also to help you break free from some taboos surrounding bladder problems and other women's issues.

My dream and the energy of this book is to share because *sharing is caring* unless it is a sexually transmitted disease, then, please, do keep it for yourself!

If this book has helped you in any way, please spread the word of its existence to as many people as you can.

So, to recap on our journey (get the selfies printed and let's do an album!):

## Adventure Highlights

- We established this book is not medical or academic but rather my opinion and a road trip with my new best friend.

- You unwrapped the presents in the free gifts section at the front of the book.

- We discovered 25 Types of cystitis and other issues that affect our bladder.

- We discovered in more depth our precious holes and how to best treat and respect them. We enjoyed 5 illustrations to help the information sink in.

- We got to know our urinary tract, what it does for us and how it can easily go wrong and why.

- We bridged the gap between clues left in our language and our bladders, precious holes and our flow.

- We took a trip down the rabbit-hole of metaphysics and now know how to apply some basic tools to help ourselves.

- We know a little on how to bridge the physical body with our metaphysical one (mental, emotional, spiritual, aura, energy).

- We explored in depth why the 25 types of cystitis happen.

- We delved into the medical world of cystitis and how medics are not experts on your bladder but how they form a critical part of our A-Team.

- We created our own **A-Team!** We learned the 16 major protocols and their sub-protocols. We now have all the tools we need to create happy bladder health, including nutritional and metaphysical. We know that by helping our bladder and following these protocols, we are essentially helping all of our body at all of our levels: bargain!

- We have met our bladder and created a positive communications link.

- We touched on the importance of forgiveness, self-love, presence, being earnest and authentic.

- We know that being sensual means able to use our senses consciously.

- We know why our choice of products we use is critical to our health. What we put on our skin is as important as what we eat. We are what we eat, drink, inhale, touch and think.

- We broke two taboos that may have been holding us back and we unchained the shackles, regaining our energy. We had a moment when I gushed about how truly amazing women are. Yep, I still love you. On the actual road-trip, this was the moment I got silly drunk (within my fulcrum limits) and emotional and we took lots of potentially embarrassing selfies. Oh, and if you don't know what I'm talking about, (maybe you were napping under your sunglasses during that part of the trip) then you need to go and re-read!

- We have lit the candle of hope and started building the community that supports and lifts us up.
  In the actual road trip, it's when we swapped details and agreed to meet up regularly over a herbal tea for catch up, support, a

good natter and perhaps a singalong or to conga with other women across the world...

- We have relaxed and enjoyed special meditations and built up a healthy morning ritual. Make sure to use your free gifts (see link at the front) and listen to me guiding you through those meditations, so that you can totally relax and be pampered.

- We have touched upon other health issues women suffer with aside from cystitis that affect our precious holes and how to potentially overcome those.

- We have an easy to follow protocol check-list to look at often so that the information really sinks in. We understand that repetition is key.

- We celebrate in the last chapter, glasses of bubbly at the ready: *chink!* Cheers!

- ***Piss to Bliss* is not just a book, it is a movement: join the flow.**

I invite you now to look back at all the chapter keypoints to remind you more fully at a glance of what we have explored together.

Do ensure that you have completed the actions steps and filled out your *Piss to Bliss Companion*, or your journal.

Glance through your workbook now and be proud of what you have accomplished on this learning curve.

Go on. I'll wait here, sipping more champagne.

Awesome! Right?

**What a trip. Thank you for being the perfect travel buddy.**

\* \* \*

Be brave and break free from any taboos, especially on bladder health, women's issues or sexual hygiene that you are still entangled with.

Be the one who stands up for self-love and bladder health.

Follow the protocols in this book that will help you heal from cystitis forever.

Tell people who are also suffering from any bladder problems where to get this book. Help them embark on their own potential healing journey. I know I have already asked you this, but you know me: repetition is key!

All that remains is for me to quietly stop writing and go our separate ways, but do remember, you are not alone.

**Cystitis is no longer a taboo.**

Please join our community on Facebook and speak out, and lastly be proud.

By reading this book, you have taken a huge leap in getting your power back and controlling your health.

You have started your self-love journey and that warms my heart and my bladder.

If I can help you from ever suffering again, then this book was worth writing. It was worth me being brave and vulnerable in sharing my personal journey with you.

If I can stand up, be brave, and help others get over cystitis, then so can you, so:

*Start spreading the news…*

Oh, come on: *sing!* I know you know the words… And I've heard your beautiful singing voice already on the road trip, right?

By reading this book and recommending it to others, you are now a part of my dream unfurling into reality. Bless you, for that.

I'm grateful that you trusted me. Now trust yourself, you have all the knowledge you need to avoid cystitis and finally be free. Enjoy.

I shall leave you, if I may, with my motto, one that keeps me on track, especially when fear comes a-knocking:

**Fortune favours the brave.**

\* \* \*

## Chapter 13 Keynotes

- There comes a time in a journey when we have to be brave and do what it takes to reach our destination. That time is now.

- Recapping is fun! What a ride we shared. Fabulous selfies too! ·

- Catchphrases are a good way to recap important information.

- You are frigging awesome, Girlfriend. You rock!

## Action! Interactive bit, it's your turn:

Write in your journal, any feelings that came up after finishing the entire book, and the answers to these questions:

1. How are you going to be brave?

2. Have you read the entire book and completed all the interactive action steps?

3. What 8 things most stood out from the book for you?

4. Have you started implementing the protocols?

5. Has this book helped you be cystitis-free or at least cystitis-less?

6. Has this book changed your life, or could it if you followed all the protocols?

7. Do you have a daughter to pass some of this valuable information onto?

8. Anything else? Go on, have a good ponder.

9. Leave an honest review of this book on Amazon and any other book platforms.

10. Propose this book at your next book-club meeting, it makes colourful debates!

11. Write down the catchphrases from this book that you like. *My favourites are*:

**List of *Piss to Bliss* catchphrases by Dr Jennifer Meyer**

- Piss to Bliss is a movement: join the flow

- Put the Yip back in Pee

- Go from Piss to Bliss

- If he refuses to be hygienic, he has no business touching you

- I had a She-Wee, not a penis

- Metaphysics is the ability to bring magic to everyday life

- You are not alone

- Keep your flaps clean!

- Treat your precious holes with reverence

- Double standards are outmoded.

- Break taboos and liberate yourself from the shackles of society

- Restore the female body with respect and honour

- Ditch the Douchebags

- Women's health issues are not dirty, shameful, or guilt-worthy: speak up

- Sensual means the ability to use your senses

- Build your Bladder A-Team

- Find Your Fulcrum

- Sharing is caring

- We vote with our money: what are you condoning?

- Command respect: you deserve it

- At least deploy some damage limitation

- Fortune Favours The Brave

- Road-Trips Rock!

- I can feel it in my waterworks

- I'm done with people beating about my bush!

- Your presence is a gift

- Repetition is key

- Linguistic Interlude!

*What are your favourite phrases from our road-trip?*

Catchphrases are important as they act as reminders of important information.

For example when you read the phrase "Linguistic Interlude" that hopefully brought up images of all the words and sentences related to our bladder or our bodies that we discussed throughout the book.

Do make a note of the phrases above and your own favourites ones from the book in your journal.

* * *

Here are my top 8 tips for bladder health:

1- Drink high-quality aloe vera gel each morning and/or before bed

2- Keep hydrated with at least 2 litres per day of still mineral/spring water

3- Wipe from front to back and clean your anus after each poo

4- If sexually active ensure to have hygienic sex (both partners clean)

5- Be authentic in all areas of your life, especially to yourself

6- Avoid inflammatory/acid-forming foods

7- Know your fulcrum

8- Value yourself and your worth, ditch any poverty belief systems

So, we have now come to the end of the last chapter. You have pondered deep questions and completed your journal with great personal insights along the way.

Truly, congratulations on your progress in your bladder health.

I thank you so much for trusting me and taking this journey together.

I welcome you to the other side: *cystitis-free living, let's make that blissful thriving.*

*Please read the following pages so you know where to go for any ongoing support.*

**I now, gently, let go of your hand.**

**I smile as I look you in the eyes: I salute you.**

:o)

PS: I still love you.

# Next Steps

Visit facebook.com/groups/497363147337943/ to join our Private Facebook Group, **The Happy Bladder Tribe**

To visit Dr Jennifer Meyer's Facebook Page:
facebook.co.uk/DrJenniferMeyer

My website, Newsletter & Blog:
drjmeyer.com
@drjennifermeyer
twitter.com/drjennifermeyer
facebook.com/DrJenniferMeyer
instagram.com/drjennifermeyer
linkedin.com/in/jennifer-meyer-5597a6196
bit.ly/2XRKLwA

Get in touch if you wish to book me for a talk on bladder health or metaphysics.

Look out for upcoming books, in case you fancy another adventure together!

To be published in 2020:

*Piss to Bliss Companion* to use as you go along the book. It would be wise to ensure you do all the exercises and read the book several times.

*Yip-Pee!* The version of *Piss to Bliss* written for girls and young teenagers.

*Yip-Pee Pal.* The companion book for *Yip-Pee.*

*Piss to Bliss* Online Course

I look forward to spending time with you in any of the above upcoming adventures.

* * *

Here are the links again to your FREE GIFTS: drjmeyer.com/free-gifts

# Acknowledgements

I feel as if I'm holding an Oscar. I launch tearfully into my gratitude for those who helped me get here… cue applause. I stand in my glamourous dress dripping in diamond jewellery as I gaze out to my audience adoringly.

I'd like to thank my parents who fought to give me life. Who supported me in all I wanted to do, no matter how bonkers. Thank you for allowing me to make my own mistakes and being there to pick up the pieces. Thank you (and Santa) for buying me the laptop I needed to write this book. You are gorgeous, I adore you.

I'm so grateful to many people. Here though, it is about those who *specifically* supported me with this book. I love you all, the list is in no particular order.

### *So, a huge thank you to:*

All at Self-Publishing School (**SPS**) for the tremendous teaching and open-hearted support, & our AAA team. I have an affiliate link to them at the start of the book. Thanks to **Chandler Bolt** and my super coaches **Gary Williams, Lisa Zelenak,** and **Sean Sumner.**

My adorable **Gagglettes**: my gorgeous friends who inspire me every day and who forgave me for being lost in my book rabbit-hole for so long. They were there for me not only during the whole writing and publishing process but during my last horrific cystitis. The daily contact helped me not feel alone whilst I was on my own in a foreign hospital fighting for my life. They cried with me, they sent me gifts, and they rejoiced with me when I was getting better. They even did a happy dance for my first

*blissful* wee. They were the first I told about the idea to write this book and have been with me all the way. Individually and as a group, they are fabulous. **So, I love you:**
**Marianne Simpson, Linet Andrea, Becki LeFevre, & Bisa Dobson.**

**Despina Panomitros,** who gave me healing and coaching and was the first to hear the phrase *From Piss to Bliss.* Her gorgeous laughter sealed the deal, I knew it was going in the title. What a road-trip! She also gave me valuable editing advice. Your continued support is magical.

**Dr Atterton** and all at my local NHS surgery, what a team!

My beautician (Hollywood star) & awesome friend, **Jelena Dreimane.**

My accountability buddy, **Rhiannon D'Averc.** We have fun and our friendship has helped build true momentum. Many gold stars and Oscar stickers light our way.

**My** *Unicorns United* **Family**, all of you at the M.T.M 2019 Breakthrough to Abundance Mexico Retreat run by Lisa Nichols & Matt Gil.

My **Dream Cheerleaderz** Accountability M.T.M Group.

**Ms M.C.Fuller,** who helped with early editing.

**Rachael Cox,** for your wonderful formatting and patience.

**Paulo Soares,** for helping me get my message out to the world.

**My village**, esp. Daphne, Christine, Barbara, Marion, Harriett & our book-club.

**My family.** English, Australian & French, especially Phainie and Nadine Duport.

My SeilenSchwester, **Sabrina Roncaldi.**

My cousin **Leanne Mitchell** for printing my first manuscript & being fabulous.

My comforting BBB's for your continuous friendship, encouragement and love: **Veronica Hufford, Janet Barclay, Shannon Milsom, Alexandra Weyman.**

All in the *Speak to Inspire Tribe* led by **Lisa Nichols,** who all sent me love and healing when I was hospitalised both abroad and at home.

My **TimeTalks** sis-tars (TT), led by my brilliant friend, **Heidi Baker,** fellow pioneers of speaking authentically & being our true selves in public. You were the first group I publically introduced this book to and your welcome and encouragement meant so much.

**Kristen Zwahlen** for our visualising fun, fairies and being my future L.A realtor.

**Juaniece Bair-Hummingbird & Trisha Dolan** for your wise open-hearted love.

My Carmen's Coffee Talk friends led by my inspiring friend **Carmen Badan:** let's manifest miracles (and helicopters).

My energy coach **Wai Cheung,** series 7 kicks some serious arse, obvs.

My darling, *Ms P.* **Philippa East,** for your encouragement and devotion to the written word that you write so elegantly, and for my first literary goddaughter.

My spiritual Goddess, **Anna Baldwin,** for Reiki and health kinesiology during my cystitis crisis, and for always being there for me. You are gorgeous.

**Adam Sheik**, Good Sir Knight, for everything, especially the humour: I.P Freely.

My Dude, **Vicki Vrint**, for unbreakable faith in me as I launch into self-publishing.

**My launch team**. You courageous peeps who believed in my book, and in me.

My beautiful boys, my cats, **Bruce and Jet**, who purred lots and sat by me encouragingly whilst I typed, putting up with late dinners and very late nights.

My cats in heaven, guides, helpers and the **universe** for always having my back.

And finally, my new friend, *You*. *YOU* were that guiding star. When I got scared about publishing my book, you kept me going, because I knew that, *you*, needed to read my story and come on that road trip!

# About The Author

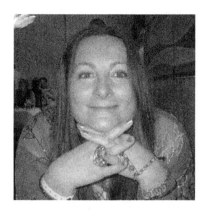

**Dr Jennifer E.L. Meyer** lives in Cambridgeshire UK with her cats. Born in the Auvergne, France, and moved to England as a child, she is French and British but considers herself *Worldwide*. Her love of languages brought her to study at Cardiff University in Wales where she graduated with a Triple Honours Batchelor of Arts Degree in French, German, Spanish, and English TEFL. She discovered a passion for Kung-Fu as she had a love for all things ancient Chinese. She experienced living abroad for her studies.

Jennifer was always holistic and aware of energy and magic. Her passion for all things metaphysical was the reason she studied shamanism, & Reiki Teachers Masters. She also has dozens of related diplomas including nutrition, aromatherapy, and tarot... She is a qualified therapist in Reiki, Massage, Hopi Ear Candling, Crystal Healing, and Life-Coaching. She trained in the benefits of aloe vera.

Whilst working in a London bank she studied part-time on her doctorate and graduated with a PhD in Metaphysics.

Jennifer created stories and poems from a young age. She invented her first children's tale on the spot when she was four-years-old, to entertain her family during a 4-hour power cut.

She enjoys writing in different genres: children's illustrated books, adult dark fiction, humorous short stories, poetry, and self-help guides.

She is now concentrating on publishing these books, as being an author finally takes priority in her career. She still coaches and will be creating online courses in several subjects. She is also a popular international speaker.

drjmeyer.com
@drjennifermeyer
twitter.com/drjennifermeyer
facebook.com/DrJenniferMeyer
instagram.com/drjennifermeyer
linkedin.com/in/jennifer-meyer-5597a6196
bit.ly/2XRKLwA

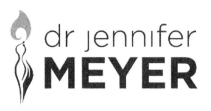

# Praise for Piss to Bliss 2019

**Dr N. Miggins, USA**

*This is such a valuable book! So many patients in my practice suffer from cystitis, ranging from mild and occasional to chronic and unrelenting. Often times standard treatment protocols failed to get them the results they were hoping for. Now I know why! Dr. Meyer does an excellent job of breaking down this complex issue into understandable and doable steps. I now feel enlightened and empowered to better serve my patients. And provide them with a resource that can impact the quality of their daily lives.*

**Shannon Milsom, UK**

*What an open and frank discussion about an important subject that most think is taboo! This book gives such a wealth of definition and practical advice to be able to help anyone who suffers "problems down below" (and those who do not) to avoid many health problems.*
*This book is so positive, speaking in modern tone and humour. It allays much of the mystery of the many conditions we don't want to talk about. Best of all anyone reading this is urged to reflect and address what they may have feared to ask and to pick up the call to action to help themselves.*

**Wes Giest, Canada**

*I loved Piss to Bliss – and I'm a guy! This book has attitude, right from the title page. Dr. Meyer does a courageous, clear, and constructive job of telling women about their bodies. She tells her own story with clarity and honesty, without inviting "poor you!" wallowing. She offers an full range of insights and solutions to issues around the topic of cystitis, and on a broader level to the challenges of being human and being female. Leaving aside the central topic of the book, Meyer gives direct and practical advice for emotional, physical, spiritual, and social health, applicable to both men and women. This book offers hope—not passive, "I wish it were otherwise" hope, but active and resourceful hope, with "you can do it!" singing between the lines. Five stars!*

## Dr B. Grossman, USA

*I laughed and cried. I was honestly surprised at how much I enjoyed this book! What a great read! Such a serious topic, an informative and broad-reaching perspective of looking at healthy urinary function, and written with a sense of humor and candor. I found myself laughing out loud AND taking notes. It's about time a book like this was made available to anyone curious about their bodies and particularly anyone who has ever had a bladder infection or cystitis. Having had chronic cystitis myself growing up, I really identified with so much of the information in this book. I was happy that the author mentioned early on that she is British because I enjoyed her accent throughout the book as well. I LOVED her explanation for the abbreviation of: "For Unlawful Carnal Knowledge". She got me thinking about taboo and language in general. I am sure I will refer back to this book, and I know I will have opportunities to refer it to others! Great read for a tough topic!*

## Julie Fleming, USA

*Piss to Bliss was delightfully helpful and fun to read!*
*It is loaded with so much information about the many urinary and vaginal issues that plague women of all ages. I am thankful to Dr. Jennifer Meyer for providing answers and antidotes I've looked to the medical community for in the past. I loved the chapter keynotes and interactive bits, as it helped seal my learning and kept me engaged. I also loved the humor it was written with that made the reading quick and enjoyable. This unconventional and refreshing self-help book is not only about the bladder, but whole body health and wellbeing! A great read!!*

## Dr Philippa East, UK

*A taboo-busting, open-hearted, informative and inspiring guide*
*I think this book will serve as an amazing resource for anyone suffering from chronic cystitis or other painful, inflammatory bladder conditions. Dr Jennifer Myer draws generously and deeply on her own experiences of severe and longstanding cystitis (now cured!) to provide a taboo-busting, open-hearted, informative and inspiring guide for fellow sufferers. The book is written with great warmth and humour, while also providing a wealth of information and insight, with detailed guidance on steps sufferers can take themselves to manage their often-debilitating symptoms and regain control of their health and lives.*

*Dr Jennifer Meyer makes it clear that this is not a medical text book, but an experience-based self-help guide, and I feel that this is potentially one of the strengths of the book. Dr Jennifer Meyer provides her own comprehensive classification system for various types of cystitis (and related conditions), presenting ways of understanding these which may be particularly helpful and revelatory to suffers who have had limited success with standard medical interventions.*

*"Piss to Bliss" is incredibly comprehensive, giving these often-dismissed or trivialised conditions such close and thoughtful consideration, chapter by chapter, and looking holistically at contributing factors and potential solutions at all levels: from the most practical hygiene tips to metaphysical principles. I particularly like the positive attitude Dr Jennifer Meyer takes, treating the journey of recovery as an exciting adventure of personal respect, throwing off the shackles of despondency and shame which can so easily shadow these difficulties. I believe this book will be life-changing for many of its readers in its gift of understanding, support and hope.*

**Dr S. Ha, Canada**

*Dr. Meyer's raw depiction of her lifelong cystitis journey is tangible and insightful. She is to be applauded for her authenticity, courage and commitment to educate others about a condition that nearly took her life. Readers of this book will cry, laugh and feel Dr. Meyer's pain and frustrations as she navigates the various health care systems that tend to treat cystitic patients rather than patients with cystitis. Her transparent and uninhibited narrative puts the "human" back into the millions of people suffering from urinary problems. I must say her captivating story and style of writing kept me engaged the whole time. I particularly liked her casual and brazen British accent leaping out of the pages, her sidebar language education and her precocious play on words. There is also just enough science and research done to back up and support her comprehensive and easy to follow protocols.*

*At its deepest core, Piss to Bliss is more than a self-help book with a clever title, it is a well written, praiseworthy acclamation to the determination of Dr. Meyer to profoundly enrich lives and to empower women/men to simple blissfulness, regardless of bladder problems, and/or other limitations. I can't wait to dive into her next book.*

# Please, Can You Help?

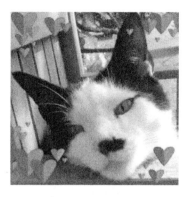

**Thank You for Reading My Book.**

**Sharing is Caring**

I really appreciate your feedback and I love hearing what you have to say.

I need your input to make the next version of this book and my future books even better.

Please leave me an honest review on Amazon, GoodReads, and Social Media.

Thanks so much!

Happy Bladder Health.

And remember it's time to put the *wee* and *yip* back in pee.

Or as the front cover says:

it's time to go from piss to bliss.

Big hugs, Jennifer xxx

Printed in Great Britain
by Amazon

67560819R00264